Praise for
Yoga Nidrā
Made Easy

'*Easy to understand and deeply practical,
this book contains everything you need to
become the nidrista that you already are!*'
CHARLIE MORLEY, BESTSELLING AUTHOR OF *WAKE UP TO SLEEP*

'*Yoga Nidra Made Easy is a beautiful journey through the
labyrinth of awakening to the power of repose. Accessible
and deep, this book full of supportive and nurturing
practices that allow you to reclaim the rest you deserve.*'
TRACEE STANLEY, AUTHOR OF *RADIANT REST* AND
EMPOWERED LIFE SELF INQUIRY ORACLE

'*This book is a gift. Its message one of profound simplicity
– that in yoga nidra, in deep rest, in standing against a
culture of constant action, we can return to ourselves.*'
JESSICA HUIE, AUTHOR OF *PURPOSE*

'*A marvellous beginners guide to the profound,
elegant practice of yoga nidra.*'
JOHN VOSLER, MULTI-LINEAGE YOGA NIDRA
EDUCATOR AND FOUNDER OF TRI-BEING

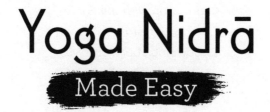

Yoga Nidrā

Made Easy

Also in the *Made Easy* series

Yoga Nidrā

Made Easy

Deep Relaxation Practices to Improve Sleep,
Relieve Stress, and Boost Energy and Creativity

UMA DINSMORE-TULI PhD
and NIRLIPTA TULI MA
Cofounders of the Yoga Nidra Network

HAY HOUSE

Carlsbad, California • New York City
London • Sydney • New Delhi

Published in the United Kingdom by:
Hay House UK Ltd, The Sixth Floor, Watson House,
54 Baker Street, London W1U 7BU
Tel: +44 (0)20 3927 7290; Fax: +44 (0)20 3927 7291
www.hayhouse.co.uk

Published in the United States of America by:
Hay House Inc., PO Box 5100, Carlsbad, CA 92018-5100
Tel: (1) 760 431 7695 or (800) 654 5126
Fax: (1) 760 431 6948 or (800) 650 5115; www.hayhouse.com

Published in Australia by:
Hay House Australia Pty Ltd, 18/36 Ralph St, Alexandria NSW 2015
Tel: (61) 2 9669 4299; Fax: (61) 2 9669 4144; www.hayhouse.com.au

Published in India by:
Hay House Publishers India, Muskaan Complex,
Plot No.3, B-2, Vasant Kunj, New Delhi 110 070
Tel: (91) 11 4176 1620; Fax: (91) 11 4176 1630; www.hayhouse.co.in

A catalogue record for this book is available from the British Library.

Tradepaper ISBN: 978-1-4019-6711-6
E-book ISBN: 978-1-78817-742-9
Audiobook ISBN: 978-1-78817-741-2

10 9 8 7 6 5 4 3 2 1

Printed in the United States of America

Interior illustrations: 14, 158 © Uma Dinsmore-Tuli; 33, 91, 95, 96, 105, 155 ©
Sivani Mata Francis; 38 © www.exoticindia.com; 62 © Nirlipta Tuli

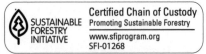

To the Divine Goddess, Nidrā Shakti Devī
who resides in all existence in the form of Sleep,
we bow to Her; we bow to Her;
we bow to Her, continually we bow, we bow.

Devī Māhātmyam (V: 23–26)

Contents

List of Yoga Nidrā Audio Recipes

Below is a list of audio recordings of the Yoga Nidrā recipes in this book. All tracks are recorded in two versions, one with a female and one with a male voice, and can be found via the 'Yoga Nidrā Made Easy' tab on the Yoga Nidrā Network website (www.yoganidranetwork.org). They will also feature on the Hay House Unlimited Audio app.

Audio track 1.0   A rhythmic yoga nidrā to remind me how to rest – Welcome home to my rested self

Audio track 2.0   Settling deeper and easier

Audio track 3.0   Ways to inner listening (#1, #2, and #3)

Audio track 4.1   Easy rhythmic journey of attention around the body #1 – Rhythmic travels by numbers

Audio track 4.2   Easy journey of attention around the body #2 – Nine encouraging reminders to embody the experience of yoga nidrā

Audio track 4.3   Easy journey of attention around the body #3 – Complete tour (108 invitations)

Audio track 5.0   Easy opposites (#1 and #2)

Audio track 6.0   Serving suggestions to connect to imaginative capacity (#1 and #2)

Audio track 7.0   Special ingredient: Keeping curious as you return to inner listening

Audio track 8.0   Externalizing recipe (#1 and #2)

Audio track 9.0   Serving suggestion – Completion

Audio tracks 10.1–10.8   Making the practice your own: Stages 1–8 Embodied knowing

Audio track 11.0   Welcoming wild nidrā

Audio track 12.0   Welcoming wordless yoga nidrā

Audio track 13.0   Yoga nidrā in the stars

Introduction

in the worlds of yoga nidrā –
at the threshold to the dream
there are people settling
their tired bones upon the earth

in the worlds of yoga nidrā –
as the thoughts and feelings ebb
there are bodies breathing
into spaces of deep quiet

in the worlds of yoga nidrā –
as the sounds are welcomed now
there are conscious sleepers
taking refuge in this rest

Welcome to your experience of yoga nidrā: an effortless state of restful being in freedom. Yoga nidrā is a horizontal meditation upon the threshold of sleep, a conscious way to rest that invites you to nourish every aspect of yourself. It may look as if absolutely nothing is happening, but the deepest of restoration is occurring.

Yoga nidrā is not just a practice, but also a form of awareness; not simply a technique, but a naturally cyclical nurturing process for entering and inhabiting restful and creative states of consciousness that are every rested human's birthright. To encounter yoga nidrā is to rest in freedom. We believe yoga nidrā is everybody's treasure, and the radical intention of this book is to liberate that treasure for you and for everyone everywhere who wants to experience natural yoga nidrā.

Just how simple are you prepared to let this be? If you can recall what it is like to have fallen asleep and woken up again, then you know how it feels to be in yoga nidrā. You can welcome this nourishing and restorative experience again, any time you like – no movement necessary, no teacher necessary, no special equipment necessary (except a timer!).

Yoga nidrā can be easy, and this book shows you how.

When we were asked to write *Yoga Nidrā Made Easy* we wondered how to squeeze 60 years of experience and 3,000 of practice into 200 pages. We asked ourselves: What is the best way to make this easy? What is the simplest way to share the gift of yoga nidrā, to make it easy to do, to make it easy to feel, to make it easy to remember?

First, we simply remind you that you have already experienced yoga nidrā. Second, we guide you to recall what you already know, by sharing the essence of yoga nidrā in the simplest words, through easy rhythmic games and recipes to help you experience this cyclical process of restoration and integration, whenever and however suits you best, in your own time, on your own terms.

Making yoga nidrā easy makes it accessible. Humans who practice yoga nidrā can rise up rested and nourished, able to be fully and freely themselves. Yoga nidrā can help people face the everyday challenges, injustices, sufferings, and joys of being human with balance, dignity, and the inner strength of deep resilience. Practicing yoga nidrā invites freedom from stress by restoring the natural rhythmic cycles that support all life. This is a vital resource for everyone. *Yoga Nidrā Made Easy* brings authentic yoga nidrā to the people now!

At your service!

We are Uma and Nirlipta, cofounders of the Yoga Nidrā Network, and we wrote this book for you. We are here to make yoga nidrā easy for you, to guide you through an effective, gradual approach to an authentic process of yogic sleep.

We set up the Yoga Nidrā Network in 2010 with the simple intention to support global practice of yoga nidrā in every mother tongue. Our network freely shares recordings in 23 languages, and we train and support teachers in the ethical facilitation of yoga nidrā. We want everyone who would like to experience yoga nidrā to have free access to expert, reliable guidance, and authentic recordings for their personal practice.

Why do we want to do this? Because we know from the direct experience of our students, our teachers, and our own – just as many millions of other people around the world know – that yoga nidrā is a powerful, radically nourishing practice that can deeply restore healthy sleep, vitality, and creativity. *Yoga Nidrā Made Easy* unleashes the liberatory processes of yoga nidrā so that you can simply and easily practice it by yourself, anywhere, anytime, without depending upon commercial recordings and trademarked methods.

Yoga Nidrā Made Easy distills the essence of our combined 60 years of yoga nidrā teaching experience and shares the benefits of this valuable process with you. There's no organization to join, no guru to worship, and no complex beliefs to adopt. There's just a simple, straightforward, nine-part cyclical process that is super easy to follow and remember. All you need is this book and a timer.

You'll learn from your own direct experience of yoga nidrā how to make this process part of your daily life, improving sleep, relieving stress, and boosting energy and creativity. We've made yoga nidrā easy for you by condensing 10 years of training Total Yoga Nidrā facilitators into the world's friendliest, simplest, and most thoroughly encouraging open invitation to make yoga nidrā your own.

Our yoga nidrā stories

We both first met yoga nidrā in 1969, when we were little children who loved, like so many small humans, to inhabit magical spaces between waking and sleeping, restful and creative places of dreams and imagination. It was not until many years later that we each independently realized that these states of being could be accessed through the practice called yoga nidrā. Uma first drifted unknowingly into the state of yoga nidrā as a four-year-old Londoner watching *Yoga for Health* on Thames Television with her mother. Inspired to create small meditative practices of yogic sleep for herself in her waking life, she used her intuitive, child-sized version of yoga nidrā to access creativity, writing poems and stories, and dreaming lucidly throughout her childhood. When Uma first met the formal practice of yoga nidrā in a yoga center in London 20 years later, she immediately recognized it as the same state of restful being through which she had channeled boundless creativity as a little girl.

North of London, at home in Luton, Nirlipta's boyhood was shaped by multiple spontaneous encounters with states of yoga nidrā. These experiences inspired his paintings and drawings, designs and decorative arts. As a young painter and art historian, he rediscovered yoga nidrā in the same London yoga center where he later met Uma. Our marriage, our family, and whole working life together are a direct result of our encounters with yoga nidrā.

Our adult meetings with yoga nidrā as a formal meditative practice reminded us both of those naturally occurring experiences we had as children, inhabiting the edges of conscious awareness, dreaming up stories and pictures. Our rediscovery led us to devote our working lives as yoga therapists and educators to the practice of yoga nidrā.

We have been exploring, defining, redefining, teaching, and sharing yoga nidrā for decades with people all over the world. Because we couldn't find a comprehensive enough textbook for our workshops and courses at the Yoga Nidrā Network, we even spent seven years researching and writing a 700-page encyclopedia of yoga nidrā. All practices and processes in this book are drawn from *Nidrā Shakti: The Power of Rest – An Illustrated Encyclopaedia of Yoga Nidrā* and from the rich resources of our Total Yoga Nidrā teacher and facilitator training manuals.[1]

What is yoga nidrā?

Although literally it can mean 'yogic sleep,' or 'sleep that is yoga,' or 'sleep caused by yoga,' or even the 'sleep of the yogis,' in fact yoga nidrā it is not a sleep but an awakening.

To speak about *doing* yoga nidrā is a contradiction, because in the state of yoga nidrā there is absolutely nothing to be done: Yoga nidrā is in fact a state of *non-doing*. All contemporary approaches to yoga nidrā are basically techniques to be practiced to access states of awareness that naturally arise *effortlessly*. You can't *do* yoga nidrā, because yoga nidrā is a state of *being*, not doing. The processes of *doing* yoga nidrā lead us into the state of *being* in yoga nidrā.

▶ *Need to know*

What is happening to my brain during yoga nidrā?

Yoga nidrā is an effortless meditation upon the cyclical processes of falling asleep. It trains us to become familiar with, and aware of, the states of consciousness leading into and out of sleep. All the brain-wave states that arise on the journey into sleep, and during sleep itself, are present in yoga nidrā, which is why it feels so relaxing. Experiences of these different states of consciousness can be partially identified by the presence of different amplitudes of electrical activity in the brain, and all these different brain-wave states (beta, alpha, theta, and delta waves) are detectable during the practice of yoga nidrā. (More on these in Chapters 10 and 11.)

Yours already

Yoga nidrā is a naturally arising state of human consciousness already experienced by everyone who has ever noticed themselves falling asleep and waking up. The threshold states of yoga nidrā already belong to us all. But, although the capacity to experience yoga nidrā exists within, many of us have forgotten how to access this naturally restful, creative state of being.

9

Some of the biggest obstacles blocking easy access to yoga nidrā are complex systems of practice owned by organizations promoting their own brands. In the competitive marketplace of the multibillion-dollar international yoga industry, many different modern yoga schools have trademarked the practice of yoga nidrā. The different brands vary in complexity, and there are some distinctions to be drawn between their methods, but they usually tend to offer around 10 steps, presented in sequence as a yoga nidrā meditation practice. There are some disagreements among the proponents of these methods as to which are the best or the most authentic.

In Chapter 2, we describe some of the most well-known trademarked methods. Essentially, despite the best efforts of corporate yoga brands to own the practice, yoga nidrā remains a *state of consciousness*, totally accessible to almost everyone. You can't truly own what people already remember within themselves, but trademarks and branded systems tend to complicate what is a natural phenomenon. In *Yoga Nidrā Made Easy*, our intention is to help you rediscover and recognize with confidence that the experience of yoga nidrā is a resource already within you, and nobody can possess that by giving it a brand name.

Yoga nidrā is a state arising within natural cyclical processes of rest, restoration, and integration that are common to humans of all ages. This is the experience of our hundreds of students and thousands of yoga nidrā colleagues around the world.

Special inquiry

Is there any research to prove that yoga nidrā works?

Yes, lots. The first research into brain-wave states in yoga nidrā was conducted in 1970, and there have been 60 studies in the past 50 years, evaluating the impact of yoga nidrā upon a wide variety of experiences, including stress, anxiety, menstrual pain, PTSD, and insomnia. The chapters have endnote references with more information, and if you want to know more, the resources section on our website, www.yoganidranetwork.org, as well as our *Nidrā Shakti: The Power of Rest – An Illustrated Encyclopaedia of Yoga Nidrā*, include listings of many research papers we have found on the subject.

Yoga nidrā is a cyclical process

In the interests of ease and accessibility, we have simplified the processes of yoga nidrā into a nine-part, cyclical process that always includes similar ingredients in the same order. We've also devised simple diagrams and memory games to make the process easy to recall.

The process is like a recipe, where elements are added to the mix every time in the same sequence to create the finished dish, which is subtly different every time. By the time you get to the end of this book, you are likely to be so familiar with the ingredients in this yoga nidrā recipe that you may be able, quite literally, to do this practice in your sleep!

Here are the nine ingredients:

1. Preparing for the start of your process of yoga nidra –
    claiming this moment for the radical act of rest.

2. Settling into your process of yoga nidrā – resourcing the
    body of rest.

3. Inner listening and/or an invitation for intuitive intention
    – choosing your flavor of yoga nidrā for now.

4. Welcoming attention around the body – journeying
    through places and spaces.

5. Playing with paradox and integration – inviting pairs of
    opposites.

6. Connecting to imaginative capacity – feeling into
    sensory and extrasensory knowing.

7. Inner listening and/or an invitation for intuitive intention
    – savoring your flavor of yoga nidrā now.

8. Externalizing awareness – preparing to complete your
    process of yoga nidrā.

9. Completing the cycle of your process – returning to
    everyday attention.

Although this sequenced list makes it look like a linear
process, the experience of yoga nidrā is essentially cyclical.
It's vital to know from the outset that each time you
practice yoga nidrā, you cycle through your own unique

process of resting, restoring, integrating, and externalizing that always brings you safely back to where you began, very likely feeling a bit better than when you started.

Each cycle of the yoga nidrā process has similar elements, but each experience of the cycle is unique to the person, time, and place of practice. Even if everyone is listening to the same practice at the same time in the same place, each individual will encounter their own personal experience of the yoga nidrā process.

This cycle of rest and integration is natural and effortless. It used to happen all the time by itself when we were children and babies. When we practice yoga nidrā, we invite ourselves to enter effortlessly arising cycles of revitalizing recuperation from which we may have become disconnected as adults. Above all, the yoga nidrā cyclical process simply, gently, and kindly circles you back home to a rediscovery of your rested self.

It can be helpful to see this process as an inner labyrinth containing all nine ingredients, as in the following illustration.

This simple yoga nidrā labyrinth is a helpful model to track our journey through the cyclical process of yoga nidrā: A gentle journey that may confuse us at moments, but which always brings us safely back out to where we began, restored by the path we have walked.[2]

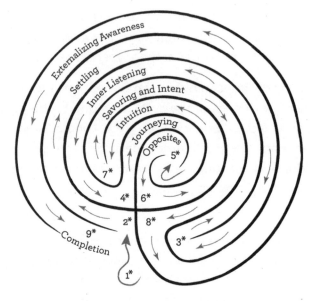

The nine-stage yoga nidrā labyrinth

To walk a labyrinth with ritual or ceremonial intent requires sacred moments of pause at the start and end of the process. Usually, a person entering a labyrinth pauses once at the threshold, once in the center, and then once again at the exit, but there may be many moments of stillness during the journey inside the labyrinth.

To walk a labyrinth, or to practice yoga nidrā, is to step momentarily outside everyday concerns with the deliberate intention to circle back into ourselves before returning to our daily life. The whole process is a threshold space in which we are free from the usual boundaries that can constrain our everyday thoughts, beliefs, and capacities.

We will return to this little labyrinth at the beginning of Chapter 10, to play a yoga nidrā memory game.

Yoga nidrā is a liminal space

The cyclical process of yoga nidrā brings us to a place and state of consciousness unlike any other because it is a liminal space. (*Liminal* is the adjective formed from the noun *limit*.) It describes the nature of a boundary, the quality of a space between spaces. Yoga nidrā is an in-between space – a threshold. In yoga nidrā, we are neither awake nor asleep, in neither one state nor another.

Many people describe their experiences of yoga nidrā's liminal, boundary state as full of paradox: 'I was asleep, but could hear just as if I was awake,' 'I could feel my body, but I wasn't able to move,' or even, 'I felt like I was fully present, but I was really somewhere else.' Yoga nidrā is an experience of being at the limits, on the edges, where one state of consciousness meets another.

A threshold, or in-between space, can be related to all the places that border it, but it is also somewhere else quite different from them. It is the place we find ourselves when we are *in transit*: We usually move through a liminal space on our way to somewhere else. Liminal spaces are not primarily intended to provide permanent accommodation. We don't usually sleep in the lobby of a hotel, we travel through it to get to the door of our own room; we don't usually stay at the entrance to a funfair, we pass through it to reach the rides we choose. As we cross the lobby of the hotel or step through the entrance of the fair, we may not be very conscious of those places in themselves; instead, we focus upon finding the way to our own room or choosing the ride that we want to enjoy.

The moment we choose to linger in these in-between places, we can encounter deep freedoms. When we choose to be present to the uncertainty of liminality, for example by resting at the threshold of sleep in yoga nidrā, we can begin to notice what was previously invisible to us, and we can recognize it for what it truly is – an openness that frees us from limits and offers up many choices and options that we could not even imagine before.

We can observe the paradox of being somewhere that is not merely 'neither one place nor another.' What was invisible or unnoticed now becomes apparent, and we can get comfortable and even discover freedom and joy in the state of uncertainty that we previously rushed to escape.

This is, initially, seemingly impossible. It is also a hugely valuable life skill, because life is full of paradoxes and pairs of opposites – grief and joy can be experienced in the same moment, and deep suffering and profound happiness can show up right on top of each other.

Through the cyclical process of yoga nidrā we can occupy the space *in between* opposites and become conscious of what was previously invisible and unnoticed in between them; we can balance on an edge that we did not even know was there.

We can inhabit these edge places, equally comfortable with chaos and order, grief and joy, or with being in neither one place nor the other. We can become conscious, still, and fully present to a state of being that was previously just an unnoticed place on our way to somewhere else. This is a paradox. It is at the heart of the yoga nidrā experience because, in yoga nidrā, we often encounter things that would seem impossible to the rational mind – like being awake and asleep at the same time – but are perfectly evident and true during the yoga nidrā state of being conscious at the threshold of sleep.

Right from the start of their first practice, many people report the sense that, 'I could hear the voice, but didn't know what it was saying.' Comments such as these reveal the presence of liminality and paradox at the same time: the sense of strangeness we might feel if we rest in a place of transit. So, when we find ourselves *consciously resting* in such a place of transit, just as we do in yoga nidrā (the threshold of sleep), we discover, sometimes to our surprise, that it is not impossible to be there at all, and more, that there can be liberty in this paradoxical space. Part of this freedom is liberation from the illusion of time. One of the key features of the cyclical process of yoga nidrā is that it can do some very strange things to our perception of time.

Yoga nidrā is an encounter with timelessness

*and all the time that ever was
is now and here in nidrā state*

After practicing yoga nidrā, practitioners often remark, 'I lost all sense of time' or 'I feel like I've been here for hours, but it's only been 20 minutes.' In the threshold place of yoga nidrā, our experience of the passage of minutes and hours often alters from everyday measurements of time. Often, that spacious expanse of time that we believe we have encountered during a yoga nidra practice – that perhaps felt like many hours – was in fact only 15 minutes.

Although some people would say these experiences distort time, in fact yoga nidrā can give us a direct encounter with the truly illusory nature of time as revealed in yoga history and philosophy. We explore this in the first chapter.

Timelessness, like every other aspect of yoga nidrā, is an immensely personal experience. In the state of yoga nidrā, each person can receive a vivid taste of reconnection to their own true nature. Nobody can define, own, or control that experience for anyone else.

We simply introduce you to the ingredients that make up the practice of yoga nidrā and show you how to combine them. We know that the recipes you cook yourself, from your chosen flavors, for your own practice, will most likely give you the taste of yoga nidrā that best suits you. That's why we have shared all our favorite yoga nidrā ingredients, along with tried and tested recipes for practice, so you can cook up the practice that's most perfect for you today, and that practice will adapt to give you what you need.

Yoga nidrā is an adaptogen

Part of the reason nobody can own or standardize the practice of yoga nidrā is because it is supremely adaptogenic. *Adaptogen* is a term used in medical herbalism, and it means that, although a medicinal plant may have multiple healing properties, only one or two will come into play in specific response to the current needs of the person receiving the herb.

As an adaptogen, yoga nidrā can be many different things to many different people. If you are basically healthy, but simply very tired, yoga nidrā may help you sleep; but if you are sick, in pain, or healing from surgery, then yoga nidrā may assist your recovery; if you are looking to boost energy, then yoga nidrā will likely leave you feeling refreshed and ready to resume activity; if you are seeking to encourage creativity or spiritual practice, then yoga nidrā may help support those endeavors.

One kind of practice, or even a single audio recording of that same practice, can have multiple, diverse, and sometimes opposite effects in many different individuals simultaneously. This is an inherent paradox, and it is a vital, key characteristic of yoga nidrā. It is literally right in the middle of the labyrinth of yoga nidrā, ingredient number five of nine.

The dynamic tension of a paradox might seem to move in two directions at the same time, just as at the center of the labyrinth. This is a productive and creative tension. We welcome paradox as one of the most important ingredients in the capacity of yoga nidrā to adapt its healing power to each person.

Standardizing the practice of yoga nidrā, to try and make it one-size-fits-all, can eradicate the potent creative ingredient of paradox. This is why we teach ways to add your own flavors to the recipes. *Yoga Nidrā Made Easy* does not prescribe a standard script, but instead embraces the creative paradox at the heart of this cyclical practice and celebrates this as part of its naturally adaptogenic nature. By acknowledging the cyclical processes of yoga nidrā, everyone is invited to reconnect with their own inherent remembrance of the natural experience of yoga nidrā and to rediscover the many ways it can support well-being: This is your invitation to get to know all the elements of this process, to make yoga nidrā your own, and to welcome whatever arises with ease. So, let's get cooking!

How to use this book

Your guide to your practice

The book is divided in two parts. Each part presents just enough theory to understand the background, balanced with sufficient practical guidance to do your own easy yoga nidrā processes.

The nine chapters in the first part of the book describe the nine ingredients of a natural yoga nidrā cycle. The second part puts the ingredients together in special yoga nidrā recipes to help you go to sleep, relieve stress, boost energy and creativity. Each chapter includes recipes to do as you read along, making it easy to feel the effects of yoga nidrā when you lie down to listen to the audio recordings.

We recommend following the practical exercises in part 1 in the order they appear to get familiar with how the cycle of yoga nidrā usually unfolds. A special nine-part process empowers you to make the practice your own, so by the time you reach the second part, you'll be confident in handling all the different ingredients in sequence. The end of the book enables you to integrate yoga nidrā in daily life. You can dive into any of the practical sections in the second part in whatever order you like.

A fresh perspective on yoga nidrā

Whether you have come across yoga nidrā very recently, or whether you are a teacher or a trainer who has already been facilitating the practice for many years, these simple recipes are intended to empower you to enjoy your own special taste of the deep nourishment of resting in yoga nidrā.

The practical ingredients and recipes in this book have all been tried and tested. They are based on techniques we have been using to train yoga nidrā teachers and facilitators since 2011. The difference here is that you are learning how to cook up a yoga nidrā *especially for yourself*, however you show up.

The book also presents the essence of the cyclical processes of yoga nidrā in the easiest and, we believe, the most authentic and powerful form possible so that you are free to practice it yourself, with or without an external guiding voice, with or without words.

Extracts from the simple rhythmic yoga nidrā at the end of this introduction are sprinkled throughout the chapters to help you easily remember the practice for yourself so that, by the end of the book, you probably won't need a script or a recording. We know it's reassuring to have words to support you, so we have made special guides to help the process, and these additional learning resources are available on our website.

Ask, don't tell!

All the yoga nidrā recipes in this book give you plenty of options. A key difference between this approach to yoga nidrā as a natural cyclical process and some of the more standard, linear ways to do the practice, is the element of genuine *choice* and *agency*.

We often tell trainees in our yoga nidrā teacher trainings 'Ask – don't tell!' It's neither kind nor helpful to *tell* people they are 'feeling relaxed' or 'tasting their bliss,' because they might well not be. Instead, it's more respectful (and ultimately more nourishing) to *ask* what is arising and adjust the ingredients accordingly.

You will notice all our ingredients and recipes include many invitations and questions so that you can gently encounter your options, and taste your way, one flavor at a time, in to cooking up the most appropriate yoga nidrā recipe for yourself every time you practice.

Rhythm, rhyme, and repetition

You'll find plenty of small songs and poems sprinkled throughout this yoga nidrā cookbook. They are special spices to enhance the flavor of the different elements, making it easier for you to remember the sequence of the process. Some of the exercises refer to the rhythmic yoga nidrā experience you will find at the end of this introduction, which is specially composed for self-practice. Repetition of the same phrases in rhythmic cycles creates a sense of anticipation and familiarity, helping you to make the practice your own so that, in the end, you don't need any words to remind you of the process.

Keeping it real: Nidrista stories

Peppered throughout the book are stories about *nidristas*. This is the word we use to describe people who practice or share yoga nidrā. All the inspiring people whose stories we tell in this book are real. Some are yoga therapy clients and yoga nidrā colleagues, some are our students, and some are teachers we have trained. We also share a few of our own adventures with yoga nidrā, to keep it real.

Need to know: Helpful guidance for your own practice

Sprinkled through the chapters you will find short answers to the many questions you may have about your own practice of yoga nidrā. The answers offer straightforward tips and hints to queries about many aspects of yoga nidrā. For example:

▶ Need to know

How long is a yoga nidrā practice?

How long is a piece of string? The length of the practice all depends on your intention for the practice and your available time to do it. An average practice for normal everyday use is usually around 15 to 20 minutes long. The briefest yoga nidrā practice could last only seven minutes, and some practices can extend to 45 or 90 minutes. Different lengths of practice have different effects because they return you to alertness from different exit points in your ultradian rhythms – the natural 90-minute cycles of your energy patterns throughout the day and night. Usually, a shorter practice is likely to leave you feeling upbeat and refreshed, while a longer practice could leave you feeling groggy or ready for sleep, unless you cycle all the way through to a full 90 minutes.

Your own recipes for your own practice

Whether you're newly arrived in the yoga nidrā world or are a seasoned yoga nidrā practitioner or facilitator, you are welcome to settle now into your own special way of being in yogic rest: This is the yoga nidrā book that gives you options and gets you 'off book.'

These recipes never *tell* you how to do this practice, instead they *ask* you to help yourself because the practice is already yours! We want to reassure you that you already know exactly what you are doing, because you've already tasted this before: Yoga nidrā is a naturally arising state of being, so you'll recognize it as a familiar experience. This book is just a helpful reminder of what you already know you can do for yourself.

A welcome gift for you – to begin here and now, just as you are

Here is our opening gift to you: your nine-minute practice of yoga nidrā to restore rhythmic cycles. You can do this right now. It's easy. Just settle back or, better still, lie down and read these yoga nidrā verses to yourself.

Notice what happens as you read. If you like, you can record this yoga nidrā later, in your own voice, or listen to an audio track of the practice in one of many different languages;[3] but please know, by the end of the book, you probably won't need a recording since you will, very likely, be able to do a whole practice of yoga nidrā all by yourself in the wordless voice of your own knowing, because yoga nidrā is easy and this book reminds you that you already knew how to do this before reading the first page. You can't *do* it wrong because there isn't anything to *do*.

A rhythmic yoga nidrā to remind me how to rest

Welcome home to my rested self

1. Preparing for the start of your process of yoga nidrā – claiming this moment for the radical act of rest.

> I take a pause to lay this body down upon the earth,
>> inviting yoga nidrā now to enter every cell.
> I lay this body down to rest. The center place is here.
> To left and right, in front and back, this body can rest now.
> The place I rest is centered in the sphere of sounds I hear.
> Above, beneath, from north and south, the sounds from east and west
>> are heard within the soundscape of this yoga nidrā space.
> Whatever sounds arising are the soundscape that I'm in.

2. Settling into your process of yoga nidrā – resourcing the body of rest.

> I notice what this skin can feel, the temperatures and touch
>> of all the clothes and covers, of the air upon the skin.
> Observing breath arriving in the nostrils as it comes,
>> observing breath departing from the nostrils as it goes.
> The settling process happening is welcomed in these bones,
>> the horizontal resting of this body here and now.

3. Inner listening and/or an inviting intuitive intention – choosing your flavor of yoga nidrā for now.

    All that I am is welcome to be.
    All that I hear is welcome to be.
    All that I feel is welcome to be.
    Just as it is.

4. Welcoming attention around the body – journeying through places and spaces.

    Making space to welcome rest in yoga nidrā here,
       attention now is traveling the paths of body-land.
    Now nourishment of rest can be received in every part.

    From crown of head to scalp it flows,
       from forehead to these brows,
          the settling body now receives the nourishment of rest.
    Between the brows, through resting eyes, the eyelids, right and left,
       between the eyes, the rest is here, and all they see is welcomed in.
    Within the ears, behind the ears, these places now can rest.
    The nostrils welcome every breath, and both the lips and tongue
       are nourished now by restfulness, are nurtured now by rest.
    The teeth and throat, the uvula, the arched roof of the mouth,
       are resting, settling into quiet, in yoga nidrā now.
    This chin is still because there is nothing to be said.

    The back of neck, the whole of spine, and both sides of the neck,
       the throat pipe now is soft within, all resting here and settling in
          to yoga nidrā now.
    Across the shoulders, down both arms, and into hands this flows.
    The yoga nidrā state is here to nourish and restore.

The palms of hands and fingertips, the spaces in between,
    the thumbs and index fingers of both hands are resting now.
On left and right, from hand to hand, the middle fingers and the
    fourth, both little fingers resting, too, and all the webbing in
    between.
The fingertips and cuticles, the nails of both these hands,
    on right and left, on left and right, the whole of both hands now
    can rest.
Every place is nurtured now by this.

Both palms and belly now can just be resting in this place.
This yoga nidrā time is now, and every breath is rest.
From belly up to chest and breasts, there is a flow of restfulness.
Within this heart, a space to be attentive to the pulse
    allows the heart and mind to be, whilst stomach receives rest,
    so centered in the navel is the nourishment of rest.

Both hips and genitals can rest, anus and pelvis, too,
    whilst all throughout the pelvic floor this rest is nurturing.
These hips and knees, these shanks and calves,
    the ankles and both feet, are welcomed in the resting place
    of yoga nidrā now.
The tops of feet, the soles and toes, the right foot and the left,
    the spaces in between the toes are settled into rest.
No need to take another step, the place to be is here.

So resting now arises in the space of every pore,
    in every hair, on every nail, through skin and flesh and bones –
    the marrow, blood, and lymph can rest.
The inner rhythms of the guts, restoring deep within
    are all in yoga nidrā time, the rhythm of deep rest.
So there is nothing to be done, but resting here and being whole.

These lungs and every single joint
   are here to rest and be restored to rhythmic cycles now.
All fluids in this body-land are restful in their flow.
They're pulsing now to rhythmic time, the yoga nidrā state.
The healing beat of vital life in every cell is nurtured deep:
   breath in, and out, and in between, now every breath can rest.
All smells and tastes, all forms and sounds, and everything that's
   known and felt, is welcomed into restfulness by yoga nidrā now.
Unnamed other places, noticed in this body now
   are nurtured here by restfulness there is no need to name:
   for every resting place is welcome, nourished, and restored
   by the space of yoga nidrā, by the act of resting here.

5.   Playing with paradox and integration – inviting pairs of opposites.

Named and unnamed, inside and out,
   from crown to soles, and toes to top,
   this body is a resting place for yoga nidrā now.

The healing beat of vital life in every cell is nurtured deep.
The parts, the whole, breath in and out, now every part can rest.
The healing beat of vital life in every space is nurtured deep,
   breath in and out, and in between, the whole of this can rest.
Now all of this, and all that is, is yoga nidrā here.

Without, within, from soles to crown, and top down to these toes,
   this body is a resting place for yoga nidrā's power.
All rhythms now can be restored, all pulse in time with life itself,
   all that is felt is nurtured now by nourishment of rest.

6.   Optional connecting to imaginative capacity – feeling into sensory and extrasensory knowing.

So just to be, as if to see this body resting now,
    so just to be, as if to glimpse a sight of this one resting here,
    so just to be, as if to feel the presence of deep rest
    restoring rhythmic cycles in the body of the earth.

The seasons of the cycles of the life within this frame
are turning now within this world of rest that is within.
This being now is welcome home, and welcomed to the ways
    that truth comes home to wisdom's way by resting here and now.
These beauty paths to wisdom's truth traverse easily,
    nurturing the welfare of this being resting here.
This simple way to freedom now is nourished by deep rest,
    and all is welcome just to be,
    and all is welcome just to rest in freedom, wisdom's way.

7. Inner listening and/or inviting intuitive intention – savoring your flavor
    of yoga nidrā now.

Restoring rhythmic cycles in the body of the earth,
    restoring rhythmic cycles in this resting body now,
    restoring rhythmic cycles in the place of restful being,
    the vital power of body's cells is dancing to this pulse,
    the beating heart of all that lives upon the body of this earth.

8. Externalizing awareness – preparing to complete your process of
    yoga nidrā.

And resting here the breath is signal to the way to be.
Four seasons of this breath are cycling now in perfect time:
breath in, breath out, breaths in between, now every breath that
    moves is felt in all the places where this body meets the earth.
All surfaces beneath me and the sounds of breathing here
    are the bridges I can cross now to return to 'every day.'

I took this pause to lay my body down upon the earth,
     invited yoga nidrā in to nurture every cell.
I laid this body down to rest beneath the sounds I heard.
Above, beneath, to left and right, the center place was here.
Throughout this pause, my body has restored the pulse of life,
     restored the rhythmic cycles of the beat of life within.
I hear my breath grow louder as a bridge to reconnect
     to the world outside this body, to the world beyond this place.

Now sounds from all directions here are welcomed in again:
above, beneath, from north and south, the sounds from east and west
     are heard beyond the soundscape of my yoga nidrā breath.
Listening out to sounds I hear, I now prepare myself
     to return to all that calls me in the world beyond my nest.

9. Completing the natural cycle of your process – returning to everyday attention.

Small movements in my fingers and my toes awaken me,
     I stretch and sigh and yawn to bring myself to waking state.
Returning now refreshed, I can resume the work I do
     to be useful and of service here to all who need me now.

This cycle of your process of yoga nidrā is now complete.
I have been reminded of the way that I can rest.
Welcome back to my rested self.

Now that you have had your first taste of yoga nidrā, let's explore the background history of the practice, from the ancient to the present.

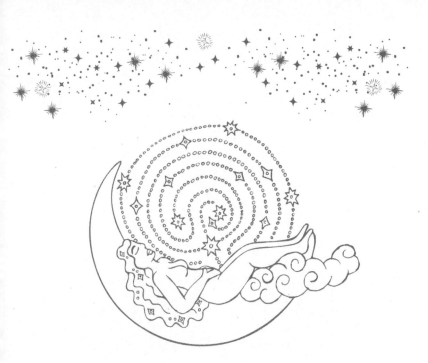

Part I

THE NINE INGREDIENTS OF YOGA NIDRĀ AND THEIR ROOTS

Chapter 1

Understanding the Roots of Yoga Nidrā

Preparing to settle into the practice

*as you begin your yoga nidrā –
gently now be here
in the space where you are resting
in this space
where you are now*

*as you begin your yoga nidrā –
let the sounds that you can hear
be welcomed
just as you are too*

Yoga nidrā is an ancient and sacred practice with many modern commercial and secular versions. This chapter explores the extraordinary history of yogic sleep and teaches you how to prepare for your own practice of yoga nidrā.

Ancient and Indigenous roots: The authentic tastes of yoga nidrā

We honor the Indigenous ancestors of modern yoga nidrā, tracking its origins in India and its journey west. Since our intention is to make yoga nidrā easy, to liberate the practice of yoga nidrā for all peoples, it is crucial at the outset to give a clear overview of the global history of the practice, including its most ancient Indian roots in the worship of the goddess.

After all, if you are going to be appreciating the flavors of the practice, it's respectful to give thanks to the people who first cultivated the ingredients and refined them with skill and insight.

Indigenous liminal dream practices have sacred origins, all arising from threshold states of consciousness very like yoga nidrā. Reverence for these in-between states is evident in many Indigenous practices of trance, dream, and ancestral connection. From the Aboriginal dreamtime stories that shape the spirituality of the native peoples of Australia, to the Toltec practices of conscious dreaming in ancient Mexico; from the Tibetan yogas of dream and sleep, to the vision-quest dream rituals of North America's First Nations and the Xhosa shaman's sleep-entry prayers for ancestral connection in Southern Africa, many earth-wisdom traditions revere the threshold places between waking, sleeping, and dreaming. These are the living, ancient traditions that first honored states of consciousness such as yoga nidrā, and they precede the modern commoditizing of yoga nidrā by thousands of years.

Every modern method of yoga nidrā meditation derives from either or both of two ancient Indian traditions: goddess worship and yoga. The first ever recorded Indian references to yoga nidrā are hymns that worship the goddess Yoga Nidrā Shakti in Indian spiritual epics that date back to the fourth century.[4] The processes for entering the creative states of yoga nidrā are right at the heart of these ancient writings. Yoga nidrā as a philosophical concept for meditation was also part of the medieval practices of Indian yoga, and it features in key texts of Indian philosophy, but the goddess Yoga Nidrā Shakti came first: she was there before the yogis and philosophers showed up.

Many organizations selling their brand of yoga nidrā have rewritten the multiple histories of the practice to place their own guru or founding teacher at the center of the origin story of the practice. The reality is, however, that no single individual has invented or rediscovered yoga nidrā, and it is neither ethical nor truthful to pretend this is the case.

In the versions of yoga nidrā history promoted by most modern yoga nidrā schools (who each, of course, have a vested interest in persuading us to believe that it is their teacher who is responsible for the rediscovery of the practice), it is rare to find any mention of the goddess Yoga Nidrā Shakti. She is the divine personification of the power of sleep in the original references to yoga nidrā in India. We need to acknowledge these roots to understand our own experiences in the process of yoga nidrā.

Yoga Nidrā is a Goddess

Yoga Nidrā Shakti Devī is praised as the divine embodiment of the power of sleep, just one of the many manifestations of the powers – the shaktis – of the goddess. There are references to Yoga Nidrā Shakti in the vast and ancient hymn to the victory of the goddess, which was first written down in the sixth century, but whose origins reach back over 10,000 years.[5] In the very first chapter of the 700 verses, all-powerful Yoga Nidrā Shakti holds the god Viṣṇu, the sustainer of the universe, under her total control.

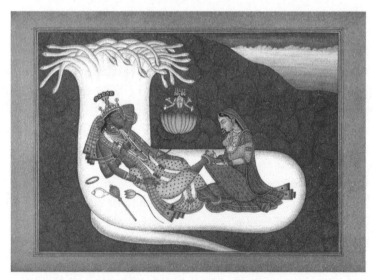

Visnu rests in the state of yoga nidrā under the control of Yoga Nidrā Shakti, whilst his consort Lakṣmi massages his feet

While he is sleeping, an enormous lotus grows up from his navel, and seated in the flower at the top is Brahma, the creative power of life itself. A pair of nasty demons threaten to devour Brahma, thereby destroying all life. Only the goddess can save him, so all the gods sing a hymn in praise of Nidrā Shakti, begging her to withdraw the power of sleep from Viṣṇu. She agrees to relinquish Viṣṇu from her control, so that he can fight the demons and save the world.

In another ancient Indian story, this time from the epic poem the Rāmāyana,[6] Yoga Nidrā Shakti uses her power to send royal princess Urmila to sleep for 14 years, much like the fairy tale of Sleeping Beauty in her palace.

The moral of these ancient tales and the many other stories about the goddess Yoga Nidrā Shakti,[7] is that sleep is a force of nature *nobody* can resist, not even princesses or gods. This is precisely why the practice of yoga nidrā is so very potent – it invites us to restore our own natural rhythms of rest and vitality, to tune in to the cycles of power that sustain all life.

There is plenty of evidence of the origins of yoga nidrā in goddess-worship practice in India. We may not literally worship Yoga Nidrā Shakti when we practice yoga nidrā (and indeed, most people practicing yoga nidrā today have never even heard of her), but even if we are not aware of her as the ancient source of this practice, whenever we lie down to do yoga nidrā, we access the state of rest, and that is a timeless power. That's why 20 minutes of yoga nidrā can *feel like* two hours of sleep (it's not, by the way, and we explain why in Chapter 11). It is also why many people feel profoundly restored, as if they have rested for a whole afternoon, when in fact they've only been in yoga nidrā for 15 minutes. It's a genuinely timeless experience.

Time traveling with yoga nidrā

Meditation on the timeless threshold of yogic sleep is described in one of the most well-known philosophical texts on yoga practice, the seventh-century *Yoga Sūtra of Patañjāli*.[8] The relationship between the four different states of consciousness is also the focus of one of the most profound expositions of Indian philosophy, the *Māṇḍukya Upaniṣad*,[9] which analyzes the experiences of waking, dreaming, sleeping, and the fourth place beyond all of these. In Chapter 13, we explore how these different states of consciousness show up in yoga nidrā, and how they can support your vitality and creativity.

The ability to remain aware while traveling freely at will between different states of consciousness is one of the aims of yoga practice. The yogins (people who practice yoga) in medieval India sought to understand the reality of concepts like time and space. They recognized that a sense of timelessness was a key characteristic of yogic sleep.

These yogins accessed yoga nidrā through a variety of yoga practices. They compiled their favored techniques in medieval yoga guidebooks. One of the most famous is the

Hatha Yoga Pradīpikā, written around 1450, which claims: 'For one who has attained yogic sleep [yoga nidrā], time becomes nonexistent.'[10]

Western influences on yoga nidrā

At the turn of the 19th century, many Western doctors and thinkers, concerned with the speed of modern life, became interested in relaxation practices to support human health and well-being. Several popular European and North American systems of relaxation developed in the 19th and 20th centuries include techniques very similar to the Indian practice of yoga nidrā.

1891 Among the earliest of Western practices similar to yoga nidrā was a series of breath-based relaxation practices presented by Massachusetts writer Annie Payson Call in her book *Power Through Repose*, which influenced key US medical doctors, including the father of Western psychology, William James.

1911 Swiss doctor Roger Vittoz published *The Teaching of Brain Control*, describing his methods for treating patients with insomnia and nervous breakdowns. Vittoz's relaxation techniques included a rotation of consciousness around the body, just like in yoga nidrā. His methods were endorsed by the English poet T. S. Eliot, who spent three months in Lausanne, Switzerland, with Vittoz while writing his seminal work *The Waste Land*.

1924 French physician Émile Coué, developed a system of relaxation with affirmations and resolutions that he called conscious auto-suggestion, which uses practices similar to yoga nidrā to create models for positive thinking.

1934 Chicago psychiatrist Edmund Jacobson devoted his entire medical career to developing muscular and mental tension-relief techniques that he called 'progressive and differential relaxation.' Jacobson first publicized these biofeedback methods in his popular book *You Must Relax!* Jacobson's methods were picked up by Indian teachers and incorporated into the hybrid of modern yoga nidrā.

1975 The science behind the benefits of relaxation went fully mainstream with the publication of the bestselling book *The Relaxation Response* by pioneering Harvard medical doctor Herbert Benson. In it, he provided the scientific proof behind the many beneficial biological and physiological changes that arise as humans relax. The global influence of Benson's and Jacobson's work was significant.

The impact of these many Western medical and scientific endorsements of relaxation as a key to human wellness was also felt in India.

The next section explores how ancient Indian roots, and more recent Western medical research into the benefits of relaxation, have been combined by contemporary yoga schools into the hybrid methods in the commercial yoga marketplace. We outline some of the most widespread current forms of yoga nidrā so you can get a sense of the range of different approaches to the practice. Being familiar with a few major modern methods will make it easier for you to navigate your way to your own special process of yoga nidrā.

The ancestry of yoga nidrā

All modern methods of yoga nidrā are hybrids between ancient Indian traditions and Western science. It is this hybrid basis from which modern yoga schools developed their own approaches to the practice of yoga nidrā. All Indian yoga schools teaching yoga nidrā have incorporated Western scientific explanations and relaxation techniques in their systems for practicing yoga nidrā.

European and North American medical investigations of relaxation were valuable to the development of modern yoga nidrā methods in India. Those Western doctors had been inspired by Indian philosophical ideas. There was two-way traffic on the path to the development of contemporary yoga nidrā.

Contemporary schools and methods of yoga nidrā

There are many different schools and methods of yoga nidrā. Of the four main approaches most popular today, three were founded by Indian teachers and one by a US psychologist: Satyananda Yoga Nidrā™ was developed by

Swami Satyananda; Swami Rama devised the yoga nidrā practice of the Himalayan Institute; Amrit Desai created the I AM Yoga Nidrā™ method of Amrit yoga nidrā; and American psychologist Richard Miller's secular iRest™ (integrative restoration) yoga nidrā method is derived from traditional Indian techniques. Our own Yoga Nidrā Network's independent, responsive, and co-creative Total Yoga Nidrā is rooted in ancient practices and draws upon the best of all the four main modern schools. There are other popular trademarked techniques deriving from these schools, including Tracee Stanley's Radiant Rest and Rod Stryker's ParaYoga™, both of which derive primarily from Swami Rama's Himalayan Institute approach; Karen Brody's Daring to Rest method and Julie Lusk's applications of yoga nidrā for stress reduction, which are both rooted in the Satyananda Yoga Nidrā™ method. (There are other popular methods derived from these schools, which are listed in the resources section.) To keep things simple, in this chapter we'll just focus on the main methods.

What are the differences between the different schools of yoga nidrā?

Across the four main yoga nidrā schools, there are more similarities than differences. It is easy to see that their distinct yoga nidrā recipes share many key ingredients. Most of them follow very similar sequences.

All methods begin with settling and drawing attention within and end with guiding awareness back out to everyday alertness. Most methods incorporate breath awareness and a statement of intention, affirmation, or resolve – sometimes referred to as a *sankalpa* – at the beginning and end of practice. (We share more about this ingredient in Chapters 3 and 7.)

Nearly all modern yoga nidrā methods also include pairs of opposite sensations, feelings, or experiences (see Chapter 5). Some methods use visualizations and imagination, and some don't, but every single form of yoga nidrā guides attention around the body, often following a particular itinerary associated with the particular school or lineage.

The distinctions between different schools are largely a result of the intentions of their founders. Schools founded by Indian monks (*swamis*) tend to focus attention on yoga nidrā as a traditional meditative spiritual practice. Founded by a psychologist, the secular form of iRest has encouraged the use of yoga nidrā for therapeutic applications as well as meditation. It is not necessary to separate the spiritual intentions of yoga nidrā from its psychological or physical benefits, but it can be helpful to clarify the primary intention of the practice, to make it easier to adapt the methods to your own individual purposes.

Recent developments

A positive outcome of this diversity of trademarked yoga nidrā methods is that between 1970 and 2010, the practice was promoted by several organizations simultaneously, which increased its popularity. By 2011, yoga nidrā had become a well-established niche practice in the yoga world, with the main schools training hundreds of teachers annually.

Although many schools have registered trademarks of their versions of yoga nidrā, it remains a naturally arising experience that is freely accessible to all humans. Those who genuinely seek to promote the benefits of yoga nidrā necessarily question the integrity of trademarking a state of consciousness.

Independence and freedom to rest

To ensure that your practice of yoga nidrā can most easily meet your current needs, we have chosen to keep the teachings of *Yoga Nidrā Made Easy* completely independent of any of the main yoga schools, and thus free from adherence to the traditions and structures of any single method of practice. This not only keeps things simpler, but it also widens the range of ingredients for your recipes of yoga nidrā, since you can choose from a variety of approaches, unlimited by the methods of any single school or teacher.

Our intention is to give you easy access to the benefits of yoga nidrā, using the most authentic means of practice. To do this, we draw directly from the ancient roots of yoga nidrā as a state of reverence for the radical power of rest and sleep. The essence of all effective practices of yoga nidrā rests in their capacity to help us rest, and the key to this natural process is in the depth of settling.

Cautionary note

While all major schools of yoga nidrā present practices of immense benefit to their many students, it is important to know there is ample evidence of abuses within some of these institutions. Here is not the place to go into details of these harmful actions, but it is crucial for anyone who puts their trust in teachers and trainers of yoga nidrā to be fully informed about the unethical behaviors of those who founded or lead the organizations with whom they are training and practicing. We draw your attention to this information in our role as independent teachers and practitioners who want to make the practice safely accessible to all.

We believe that yoga nidrā is everybody's treasure, and we want you to be able to benefit from it by practicing safely, easily, and on your own terms. We have published a compilation of evidence, including links to court papers, statements, and investigations conducted into a variety of unethical acts perpetrated by prominent teachers within all four main schools.[11] We have also published various statements in defense of the practice of yoga nidrā, so if you are interested to know more, we invite you to read these statements.[12]

You too have ancient roots!

Just as the ancient, Indigenous histories of yoga nidrā are intertwined with all the modern methods and forms, you, too, can rediscover the ancient roots of this practice already within you right now.

An ancestry of exhaustion

Remember that, fundamentally, yoga nidrā is the conscious cultivation of naturally arising states of human consciousness. Once upon a time, your ancestors knew this. They carried it in their bones, honoring natural cycles of rest, repair, and regeneration. Then, perhaps, they learned to override these cyclical urges to rest, losing track of natural capacities to hover at the edges of sleep and access creative dream insights. Perhaps, too, as history played out, these tired ancestors were displaced, uprooted, or labored too hard in others' lands and factories, ground exhausted into early deaths. Maybe they forgot how to rest, or maybe rest was brutally denied to them, and maybe their fatigue lives even now within you.

We are all still part of the rhythms of this planet, and yoga nidrā is a route back to reconnection. Very likely, you may remember, at a cellular level, how it feels to rest in yoga nidrā. You may very well recall how this feels, and you probably have already encountered this experience many times. It is your birthright to reclaim and inhabit this remarkable way of being in between, of simply welcoming this liminal place of deep rest.

The easiest way to connect to the experience of yoga nidrā is to *rediscover* that you already know what it is and to remember that you have already felt and recognized what it is like to be in space of yoga nidrā because – and we can't emphasize this enough – you have already been there.

Perhaps you encountered yoga nidrā in your childhood, maybe as you drifted in your dreams, probably in the effortless welcome of flashes of inspiration or during meditative moments. In all these moments and at all these times, the capacity to rest in the practice of yoga nidrā has been within you.

Nidrista story: Rest is resistance!

Radical restfulness is at the heart of the Nap Ministry, an Atlanta-based collective that promotes public acts of radical rest. Founder Tricia 'the Nap Bishop' Hersey is a big fan of yoga nidrā. She says the Nap Ministry 'is a social justice movement and we have never identified ourselves as being a part of the wellness industry. We are deeply committed to dismantling white supremacy and capitalism by using rest as the foundation for this disruption. We believe rest is a spiritual practice, a racial justice issue and a social justice issue. I began... to honor my body via rest for the rest [my Ancestors] were never able to embody, due to slavery and capitalism. This is about more than naps.'[13] (Learn more about the Nap Ministry in the resources section at the end of the book.)

The good news is that even though you may have consciously forgotten all about it, this capacity is still there now, and this book helps you to rediscover this practice, and to make it your own, free of any scripts, free of anybody else's voice, free to rediscover this spacious ease within yourself.

All you need to do to take the first step is to make time and space to welcome the nourishing taste of this practice within you – so let's get cooking!

Chapter 2

Settling into Your Natural Process of Yoga Nidrā

Resourcing the body of rest

*when we begin with settling
in yoga nidrā land –
we feel the earth beneath our bones
we rest in liminality –
and every place is where we are*

Now that we've built up an understanding of the roots of yoga nidrā and its modern methods, let's talk about making your own nidrā nest, learning how to settle, and (most importantly) knowing how to leave the process refreshed and ready for life.

Settling is the most important ingredient of yoga nidrā. It is always the first part of every recipe, and sometimes it is a very significant proportion of the entire process. This chapter explores some of the most effective methods so that every time you practice yoga nidrā you can settle completely to receive the benefits.

▶ *Need to know*

I'm pregnant. Can I still practice yoga nidrā?

Yes. The tiredness, physical discomforts, and emotional challenges of all stages of pregnancy can be relieved through the practice of yoga nidrā. The key challenge is getting comfortable enough to practice. Well-propped side-lying is recommended. Women and pregnant people who have become familiar with the practice of yoga nidrā during gestation often find that the state of yoga nidrā can support their experiences of the processes of labor and birth.

Your yoga nidrā kit

1. You'll need a timer – to keep track of timelessness. You can use a cook's timer for your yoga nidrā recipes or even an alarm clock. You can use the alarm on your phone, so long as you pick a special ringtone for your yoga nidrā wake-ups. Make sure to put the phone on 'Airplane Mode' so you don't get pinged during your practice.

2. All the practices in the book are available as audio tracks for you to access on our website, but we strongly recommend that you also make recordings for yourself. It doesn't have to be fancy. Use a simple

voice-memo function to make audio recordings of the nidrā invitations, or send yourself cues in your favorite messaging app on a single conversation thread with all your favorite recordings in one place. Be sure to choose one without a time limit so you don't get cut off.

3. Headphones are optional. If you use them, pick a style that is comfortable when you are lying down. Check that they don't stick into the back of your head. Sometimes ear buds are easier to manage.

Essential ingredients: Time and space to rest

Preparing to settle into the practice

Start with the following three steps:

1. Ask yourself, 'Do I have time for yoga nidrā in my life?'

    If the answer is, 'No, not right now,' then ask the crucial follow-through question: 'Can I *make* time for yoga nidrā in my life?' Then you can honestly answer yes! After all, here you are reading this book, so you have *already* made the time you need. Well done. The time it takes to read the exercises in this book is all the time you need to practice yoga nidrā.

2. Ask yourself, 'Do I have *space* to rest in my life?'

    If the answer is, 'No, not right now,' no worries. You don't need to have the perfect 'forever' space this very moment. All you need to do today is to find a space good enough just for now, and that will be perfect.

You could use your bed or sleeping space as long as you make some small change to signal to yourself that this is not the same as 'going to bed to go to sleep' but that you are using the bed to *rest in yoga nidrā*. It doesn't need to be a big change, just something significant enough to make it feel a bit different, like pointing your head the opposite way. Even lying on the floor beside the bed can be enough of a change. See what works for you.

You might even lie down in the bathroom or the kitchen, or under your desk. Perhaps you could tilt back the office chair to feel more rested, or pop your feet up on the desk. Nowhere is off limits, so long as you can get 15 minutes without disturbance.

Some people rest in a vehicle: either lying down on the back seat, with knees bent and feet on the seat, or reclining the driver or passenger seat. If you are going to practice in a vehicle, make sure you park somewhere safe, and maybe lock doors and windows.

It's nice to have the space to yourself, but even this is not strictly necessary. So long as you can close your eyes, then you can quietly practice anywhere, even if there are other people about. This requires a bit of an advanced skill, so to begin, we recommend finding a place where you can practice in the same spot by yourself each time. Make it your 'nidrā nest.' With practice, you can learn to use the way you feel in the external space of your nidrā nest to cultivate your own capacity to make a restful space *within* you.

*reverence for restfulness will powerfully repay
investment in your restedness – creative interest rates.*

3.   Dedicate your space to your practice.

> Congratulations if your answers to questions 1 and 2 are 'Yes, I am already making time for this, and I can find some small corner of my working or living space to rest.' Now is the time to dedicate this space to your practice of yoga nidrā. Do whatever you need to make your nidrā nest welcoming. Simply knowing that you have made this little place for yourself to rest is very profound, because it signals that you are *making space to rest*. This is a radical act of resistance to the powerful urge to be always doing, so don't underestimate the impact it can have.

> First, make sure the space is clean and dry and warm enough for you to rest still long enough for your body to settle. Check that there is enough space to stretch your arms above your head and out to the sides. You don't need to lie flat with your legs straight out. Some people find it more comfortable to bend their knees, with their feet flat on the surface beneath, about hip-width apart. We'll be exploring upgrades to your comfort levels in the next chapter, so for now, just keep it simple.

> Be sure you have enough support beneath your body to be comfortable to rest – a folded blanket, mat, rug, yoga mat, or a sheepskin – whatever you have to hand, even a coat or shawl can give sufficient softness and support. You don't need a lot because some of the practices are only 10 or 15 minutes, but it's good to know you could continue to rest for longer if you need to. If you have time once you are settled, you could listen again to the first audio track.

▶ *Need to know*

What time of day is best to practice yoga nidrā?

Whatever time that you have available. Any time at all can be helpful, and it is more beneficial to find a moment to do the practice than to choose not to do it because it's not the usual or the 'right' time. Yoga nidrā works very well at many different moments during the day or night. In fact, many people feel that practicing first thing in the morning is the very best start to the day.

Key ingredients for settling in

1. Find time and space to make your own cozy nest for your yoga nidrā practice and know there is nothing to achieve.

2. Ask yourself, 'Am I cozy enough (especially my feet)?' Bear in mind your body temperature drops a few degrees during yoga nidrā, so be sure to have warm enough covers to prevent getting chilled. If you don't feel like you need the cover at the beginning, then just have it handy so you can snuggle under it later.

3. Make sure your feet are warm enough before you start. Have you ever tried to get to sleep when your feet are cold? If so, then you'll know it's almost impossible to rest with chilly toes. Some people find that a special pair of nidrā socks is a nice touch – whatever it takes, just so long as your toes are cozy.

4. A hat can also be helpful if you are in a drafty place, especially to keep your ears warm. Although some people deliberately like their hands outside the covers, it can be comforting to rest your hands on your body beneath the blanket. (More on posture in the next chapter, but for now just rest your hands wherever it feels natural and easy.)

5. Minimize visual disturbance. The easiest way is simply to close your eyes. If you don't feel comfortable doing this, it's fine just to look down and rest the eyes, or to open them briefly every so often. If it's possible, dim the lights, or close the curtains or blinds. If you are practicing outside, rest in the shade. Some people like to use a special eye pillow or an eye mask,[14] but a scarf is fine. You could simply pull your hat, or your hair, over your eyes.

Nidrista story: When relaxing is stressful

Mike was recommended to practice yoga nidrā because he experienced high anxiety, frequent splitting headaches, and irritable bowel syndrome. Much against his will, Mike's girlfriend brought him to a Total Yoga Nidrā workshop. He was very reluctant to come. 'Every time I hear the word "relax," it makes me more stressed. It actually gives me a headache.' To his surprise, he settled deeply into the first practice, and after half an hour, he woke up with a massive smile. 'What a relief! You didn't tell me to relax,' he said. 'My headache is gone, and my belly feels more comfortable. I felt like you gave me permission to chill. Nobody told me to do anything.'

It's very common for instructors to tell us to relax when we begin a yoga nidrā practice. In fact, it's probably the most repeatedly issued instruction in most schools of yoga nidrā. But being told that you are 'relaxed' or being given an instruction to 'just relax' does not necessarily help you get settled. It can have the opposite effect.

If you are already feeling unsettled or stressed, being ordered to relax is not helpful. It is more effective to ask some simple questions about the sensations of settling down. This inquiring approach tends to be much more settling than simply giving instructions.

As you read the following series of simple questions and invitations, see what happens. How do you respond to these inquiries and gentle encouragements?

▶ Need to know

Is yoga nidrā suitable for teenagers?

Sometimes. It depends on the willingness of the teens to engage with the practice and on the nature of the recording or the facilitator. Short (20 to 30 minute), standard recordings made for adults can be suitable for teens, but the standard position of lying flat on the back with palms up and out at the sides is not always suitable for teenagers. Many facilitators of yoga nidrā for teens observe that a comfortably propped side-lying or fetal curl position is more favored.

Can children practice yoga nidrā?

Yes. Depending on the age of the child, shorter practices may be more suitable. More playful, light-hearted approaches can work best. Narrative structures for yoga nidrā and the invitation for fantasy and invention can be welcomed by children practicing yoga nidrā.

Key ingredients: Inquiries to welcome settling through the cycles of the breath

Next time you lie down to practice yoga nidrā, invite some of these inquiries to arise to support your settling processes. You can simply read and breathe, or if you like, listen to audio track 2.0 for this chapter (see listing on page 1).

1. What can I do to let this resting body become even a teeny-tiny bit more comfortable?

2. How about the breath? Can I let it travel freely through the nostrils, in its own sweet time?

3. Can I notice how far into this body the breath travels on the inhalation, and how far out of the body it travels on the exhalation?

4. What about the places in between the in-breath and the out-breath? Can I notice these places, too, in the journeys of the breath? Is the breath still in these places, or is it moving? How about welcoming these turning places in the breath?

5. How about the exhales? How do they feel? How about counting them? Maybe just noticing *nine* easy out-breaths, like this – counting down from nine to zero, knowing I can stop whenever I like, or I can repeat this process as often as I need to settle this body more deeply into rest.

6. Encouraging gentle reminder: There is nothing more that I need to be doing right now. It is more than enough simply to be here, breathing and noticing the processes of settling.

7. What if stillness comes? How can I welcome that? I know that I can settle deeper into the restfulness it brings.

8. What if the desire for movement arises? It is likely to pass. But if it persists, that will be because the body is calling for attention, so if I make

the movement this resting body calls for, then stillness is more likely to return.

9. Encouraging gentle reminder: All movements of this body are welcome. Every wriggle or cough, every fidget or sneeze, any movements that may arise can be welcomed with kindness as a way to settle back into stillness.

▶ Need to know

I heard yoga nidrā could trigger previous trauma.
Is that true?

All yoga nidrā does not necessarily trigger trauma. It will depend on the nature of your trauma, the way you manage it in everyday life, and the nature of the yoga nidrā practice you are doing. There is good research to show that yoga nidrā can be helpful for some people experiencing PTSD.[15] Invitational practices that offer genuine agency to practitioners by explicitly inviting you to negotiate the needs you have for safety and security at the start of the practice are more likely to feel 'safe,' whereas prescriptive practices that deny agency are more likely to trigger trauma. Yoga nidrā that you do for yourself, and yoga nidrā delivered in permissive language, is usually far less likely to trigger trauma than prescriptive, bossy scripts. Having options to choose where you put your attention, or what you are invited to 'see' or feel is very different from being told precisely what to do. A vital aspect of trauma-informed yoga nidrā is to keep the cues 'within the room' and to notice easily observable sensations such as your own breath or the connection between the body and the surface beneath. If trauma is triggered, return to noticing these sensations to externalize your awareness.

Settling and settling deeper

The following exercises teach you how to deepen your settling into your practice of yoga nidrā through sensory awareness, guiding attention around the body, and reviewing the day. They can all be practiced in your yoga nidrā nest or in bed at night as you go to sleep.

Remember to set your timer for 20 minutes if you want to wake up at the end.

Key ingredients: Upgrading your nest – Changing position and using props

Most images of people doing yoga nidrā show them flat on their backs on a mat or a hard floor, without any pillow, their palms facing up to the sky. This may be a comfortable way for you to practice, but if it's not, there are some very easy adjustments you can make to the traditional flat-on-your-back pose, known as the *corpse* in yoga.

First, you can rest the palms of your hands on your belly or anywhere else that feels comforting; second, you can upgrade comfort levels by adding simple props.

Here are our top three tips for easy propping to increase your comfort for daytime or nighttime practice:

1. Pop a pillow or a folded blanket beneath your head. Tucking the edge of the pillow under the tops of your shoulders can help you to settle.

2. Support your thighs or knees. A pillow, bolster, or rolled blanket can change the angle of your lower back so it's more comfortable. The closer you bring the support to your bum, the easier it will feel on your lower back.

3. Try resting on your side if you are uncomfortable on your back. To do this easily, you will need a thicker pillow to fill the space between your shoulder and ear. You'll also need additional support under you so your hipbones don't dig into the surface beneath, plus support under the upper leg, or between the two knees.

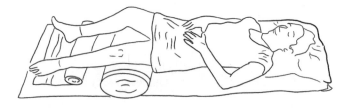

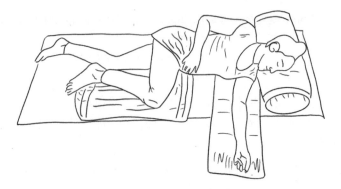

Support and props can increase your comfort

▶ *Need to know*

I have back pain/a balance disorder/respiratory difficulties, and I cannot lie flat on my back; how can I settle to practice yoga nidrā?

It is not necessary to lie flat on your back to practice yoga nidrā. If you have back pain or other medical reasons that prohibit you from lying on your back, there are many other positions you can choose. A simple solution to alleviate back pain in resting positions is to bend the knees and have the soles of your feet on the floor, or to place support under the thighs (see above). Resting your calves or feet on a chair or bed, or practicing close to a wall with knees bent and soles of the feet on the wall can also help bring more comfort to the lower back. Alternatively, rest on your side or belly. The most important thing is to be comfortable, and to support the position you choose in any way that enables you to rest easily.

Settling deeper to deepen the settling

Settling is the primary ingredient of yoga nidrā and of good sleep. Without sufficient settling, you simply can't do the practice, and you certainly can't sleep when you are unsettled.

When we're training yoga nidrā teachers, we tell them that they can never spend too much time helping people to settle. It is only when we are well settled that the rest of the practice flows smoothly. So let's take basic settling a little deeper.

▶ Need to know

Do I need to close my eyes to practice yoga nidrā?

No. If you feel more comfortable with your eyes open, then keep the lids relaxed and the gaze softly focused. The main reason for closing the eyes is to bring attention within, reduce distraction, and relax. If closing the eyes does not help you to relax, then leave them open. Knowing that it is OK to have eyes open or closed sometimes enables us to feel more comfortable closing them later in the practice. It is vital, however, for the facilitator to keep their eyes wide open to be able to mind the space for practitioners and to see the responses of the people for whom they are facilitating yoga nidrā. If the facilitator closes their eyes, then they cannot see the practitioners and are thus unable to hold a secure space for the people whose safety is their responsibility.

Recipe for settling deeper and easier

As you start to get comfortable, encourage yourself with the following invitations and inquiries. You can read them as you settle, listen to a recording of your own voice, or tune in to audio track 2.0 (see listing on page 1.)

1. What happens now that I have paused my previous activities, now that I am just lying down, preparing to welcome some stillness into this body? What do I notice?

2. What is happening to these lungs, this heart, and the rest of this body now that it has stopped being vertical and has become horizontal?

3. What physical posture suits the needs of this resting body today? Is it more comfortable right now to rest with this spine on the surface beneath, or to turn to rest along the side, or on the belly, or would it be easier to recline, propped up?

4. Encouraging gentle reminder: I give myself this time and space. I choose to be here and now. There is nowhere else I need to go to right now. In this moment, I find myself to be in exactly the right place, at the right time, with all the right things/people/creatures/plants around me.

5. What support is available to me right now: Would I feel more comfortable with a pillow or cushion under the back of my head, knees, and/or thighs?

6. Shall I rest the palms of these hands upon the belly or the heart, or rest them by the sides, palms up or down? What feels easiest now?

7. Encouraging gentle reminder: 'I can befriend myself in this moment. Whether or not it is easy to get comfortable, I simply take as much time as I need to get settled.'

8. Does it feel easy to close my eyes, or shall I simply let them rest?

9. Encouraging gentle reminder: 'This is my practice of yoga nidrā, and I cannot do it wrong, because there's nothing to do.'

When you are a bit more settled, use these invitations to settle deeper, to give away the weight of the body to the surface beneath.

10. How about if I just notice now all those places where this body has contact with the surfaces upon which it is resting?

11. How can I let more of the whole of this body be held by the surface beneath?

12. Can I transfer the weight from this body to the surfaces beneath it?

13. What happens to this resting body now if I let out a big sigh?

14. How can the sound of that sigh and the feeling of this breath enable me to give the weight of this body down into the surface beneath, through all the points where I can feel the meeting places between the body and the surface beneath?

15. If I sigh and give away the weight of the body with that awareness, does this body feel as if it has any more contact with the surface beneath than before?

16. After this breath, are there any parts left feeling unsupported in this position, or shall I release another three exhalations?

17. How about I let out another three exhalations, knowing I can repeat this process as often as I need to settle this body into rest?

18. Encouraging gentle reminder: The whole of this body is welcome to rest now. Every drop of blood and every cell are welcome to rest.

Welcoming the input of the senses: Trios of inquiry

Once you have settled the physical body, it is often helpful to introduce a further element of even deeper settling by gently welcoming all sensory input. This is particularly important if you are trying to get to sleep or practicing in a noisy place.

Hearing

1. What are the farthest-away sounds that I can hear?

2. In the great circle of sound surrounding this body now, what is the quietest sound at the center?

3. Encouraging gentle reminder: There will always be sounds. Wherever and whenever resting happens, there will always be sounds. The sweeter

the welcome for all the sounds that are present, the deeper the settling into the experience of yoga nidrā.

Touch

1. This air that touches the skin of the eyelids, is it moving or still? How does this air feel now upon the cheeks and the lips?

2. What is the temperature of the air entering these nostrils, and is it different from the air leaving the nostrils?

3. Encouraging gentle reminder: 'All temperatures and textures detectable on the whole of the skin are welcome.'

Sight

1. How can these eyes rest now in their sockets?

2. What is visible right now through these closed or resting eyelids?

3. Encouraging gentle reminder: All that can be seen behind these closed or resting eyes is welcomed – lights or colors or nothing at all.

Taste

1. What needs to happen to this tongue so that it can rest quietly on the floor of the mouth?

2. How much saliva is present inside the mouth now, and what can I taste? Is sweetness or bitterness present? Or sour tastes? Anything salty or astringent?

3. Encouraging gentle reminder: 'All these taste sensations that are detectable, from the root to the tip of the tongue, I notice them all. Just here.'

Smell

1. How is the breath moving in and out through these resting nostrils?

2. What odors and aromas are present on the breath inside this nose?

3. Encouraging gentle reminder: 'The whole of the weight of this body is welcomed and held by the earth beneath the surface beneath.'

No need to rush

To begin with, it can take a long time to settle, and a long time to come around. In time and with practice, you will be able to drop into a settled place more rapidly, wherever you are, and it will be easy to return to alertness. Sometimes it can be as simple as saying, 'Now, get ready for the practice of yoga nidrā,' and you will be able to get settled without any real need for further instruction. As you practice coming into and out of yoga nidrā, you'll get more familiar with the entry and exit processes. To cue the settling process, it's helpful to use similar phrases each time. If you don't feel settled at the end, simply go back to the start and repeat the cycle as many times as you need.

Remember this is your practice of yoga nidrā, and you can't do it wrong because there is nothing to do!

Recipe for rhythmic settling

The first two verses of the rhythmic yoga nidrā song at the end of the introduction (page 26) is one of our favorite ways to begin a yoga nidrā practice. Settle back now and invite your body to rest as you return to the song, reread those words, and rest in your nidrā nest.

Test your nest

Now that you've made time and found space, try out audio track 1.0 'A rhythmic yoga nidrā to remind me how to rest' in your nest. (See listing on page 1).

This is just a test run to see how it feels, so there's no pressure to dive deep. But first, be sure you know how to exit from the practice at the end. (See the following recipe.)

Completing the natural cycle of your yoga nidrā process

A cozy nidrā nest can be so comfortable that, once you have lain down in it, you often don't want to get back up again.

Since part of the point of doing yoga nidrā is to enhance your vitality, then it's just as important to be able to exit from the nest as it is to settle into it. In the labyrinth of yoga nidrā, both these processes take around the same amount of time.

You'll find more detailed exit strategies, including the use of chocolate, in Chapter 9, but here are some to get you started.

Nine key ingredients for yoga nidrā exits

1. Lightly touch the tip of your right thumb to the tip of each finger in turn on the right hand; lightly touch the tip of the left thumb to the tip of each finger in turn on the left hand; count all fingers.

2. Tuck your thumbs into the palm of each hand, curling fingers around thumbs to make tight little fists, and then slowly uncurl all fingers and thumbs, stretching out both hands very wide; alternating between stretched out hands and tight little fists on both hands at the same time.

3. Make spirals with your tongue inside your mouth and lick your lips.

4. Yawn huge yawns, with your jaws wide open, as noisy as you like, then screw up your lips and face into the middle of your face; alternate the screwed-up face with the big stretchy yawns.

5. Massage and pinch your cheeks.

6. Place your hands over your ears, pinch the rim of each ear, fold the ear flaps over and back, and tug the lobes of both ears.

7. Tap, rub, or scratch your scalp with your fingertips, and/or gently tug your hair.

8. Open your eyes, turn your head, and slowly look around the room/space in all directions.

9. Look at yourself and your surroundings; notice the colors of your clothes and covers; spot random stuff: 'Can I see three red things? Or three yellow things?'

When you have done whatever you need to awaken, take a stretch and repeat to yourself three times: 'This practice of yoga nidrā is now complete.'

It's important to be sure that the practice is over so you can be fully awake as you head back into your daily activities.

▶ Need to know

I hear yoga nidrā is just like a good afternoon nap.
Is that true?

Yoga nidrā works very well for that middle of the afternoon slump that many people commonly experience between 3 p.m. and 4 p.m. It can be very refreshing at this time to take 20 minutes or half an hour for yoga nidrā. Even a 10-minute practice at this time can be very refreshing, because the rhythms of most people's energies at this time dip very naturally and rapidly into resting states. Of course, this is not the only time of day that's good for practice – it all depends on the time available to you, and the rhythms of your day.

Special recipe: Palming

Palming is one of the simplest ways to externalize your awareness effectively so that you can return to your life feeling refreshed and alert. There are lots of other ways to do this (and we explore these in greater detail in Chapters 8 and 9), but palming is such a special ingredient that we wanted you to taste it right at the start.

1. At the end of the practice keep your eyes closed.

2. Bring the palms of your hands together and rub them until they get warm.

3. Place the palms over your closed eyelids so the skin of the palms is touching the eye sockets, and then slowly open your eyes into the darkness.

4. If it isn't totally dark, then adjust the hands.

5. Look into the darkness.

6. Slowly open the fingers to let the light come back to the eyes.

7. Slowly remove the palms from the eyes and welcome in a world of light and color.

8. Welcome back to waking reality.

9. Stretch and wriggle in your nest before you roll over to the side and sit up.

Now that you've had a taste of how delicious it feels to settle yourself into yoga nidrā and learned the basics of how to exit effectively, we can dive deeper into the other elements of the practice itself.

Chapter 3

Inner Listening and an Invitation for Intuitive Attention

Discovering the taste of your yoga nidrā for now

*as we rest in yoga nidrā let us listen to our hearts –
cultivating a deep refuge here by hearing what's within
in this state of yoga nidrā may we rest in openness –
empowered now to welcome all that is
and all we are –
we welcome intuition's gifts
our treasures rest within*

In the natural, cyclical process of yoga nidrā, once you have taken time to prepare and to settle, the next ingredient is a space for inner listening. This same space also arises on the way out of the practice. It is ingredient number three as well as seven.

It is easy to grasp the difference between the two versions of the same processes of inner listening, intentions, and/ or an invitation for intuition. They define the flavor of each individual practice of yoga nidrā. The first time you meet this ingredient, you simply taste it, whereas the second time it shows up – after you have completed the cycle of practice – you are ready to savor its flavor because it has been imbued or marinated with your natural process of yoga nidrā. We explore it again in Chapter 7, where we reflect upon the power of returning to your inner listening and intentions *after* you have been resting in the space of yoga nidrā for a while.

This chapter explores your options with this ingredient the first time you taste it, and empowers you to choose whether you would like your natural process of yoga nidrā to be guided by a specific intention, or whether it is more appropriate for you to rest in a receptive space of simply being. Both are possible at this stage in your practice.

Often, at this point in traditional forms of yoga nidrā practice, the instructor will tell us to repeat an affirmation or resolution three times. This affirmation is often referred to as *sankalpa*, a Sanskrit word with a very rich history. It is often mistakenly translated as a 'resolve,' but carries many deeper meanings, including intuitive arising of a heartfelt calling, or soul's purpose, which is why we describe this potent ingredient as 'inner listening, intentions, and/or an invitation for intuition.'[16]

▶ *Need to know*

Do I need to have resolution or statement of intent (a sankalpa) to practice yoga nidrā?

No. The origins of the practice do not include statements of specific intent for entering the state of yoga nidrā, and it is not necessary to affirm a resolve to experience yoga nidrā. It is perfectly possible and very effective to include such affirmations or resolutions near the start and end of the practice. Many contemporary yoga nidrā schools integrate statements of intent within their methods, so it may feel like necessity to include such affirmations – but it isn't. Although it may seem like an integral part of the purpose of the practice, it is not a crucial part of the experience of yoga nidrā. In fact, it is entirely optional for practitioners to choose whether to include a resolution in certain practices of yoga nidrā.

Why is this ingredient included at this point in the process?

This space can be used for setting intentions, inviting intuitive intentions, or becoming free from intentions. As we practice yoga nidrā, it is helpful to explore all these experiences. They all have value. Which one you choose depends largely on your time and stage of life. It is not necessary to stick to the same intention forever. Many people find that their intentions manifest, and then they set that focus aside and await the arrival of the next wave of intuitive guidance.

Please know that the context of yoga nidrā can potentize the process of setting intentions. Be very careful what you ask for.

Nidrista story: Using yoga nidrā to succeed

Dave used focused intention in yoga nidrā to achieve his aim of qualifying as a free-diving instructor. Free diving is a form of diving that relies on breath-holding until resurfacing. Free divers essentially aim to calm or soothe the breath reflex when diving to increase the amount of time they may spend underwater on one breath. Training involves a visceral conversation between the consciousness of the diver and their nervous system. 'I worked with the yoga nidrā system I learned in my nidrā teacher training, and I used the intention "calm dive" to progress through my certification exams,' explained Dave. 'Each level required a deeper dive, a more challenging rescue, and a longer breath-hold. As I progressed through the various levels, I used my teacher's methods and began practicing yoga nidrā with this intention prior to each challenge, repeating my sankalpa *three times near the start of the practice and then again near the end.' Dave triumphed in his instructor examinations, completing his certification in record time.*

Whether you hold a clear intention for a specific achievement, or welcome intuitive intentions to arise, or wish to remain in a space of freedom from intention, this yoga nidrā ingredient brings all these flavors into the practice recipe.

It is equally possible simply to rest in sublime freedom from all intentions. Ultimately, an effortless arising of intuitive guidance may be welcomed through the process of inner listening so that the purpose unfolding in our lives is the same as the experience of letting go into the flow of life.

Three serving suggestions for ingredient 3

Hear the voice of your own inner teacher as you read these invitations, or listen to audio track 3.0 (see listing on page 1).

Ways to inner listening #1 – Simply being

As you settle into this process of yoga nidrā, how about simply being without any expectation or anticipation? Using the same familiar phrases can encourage easily dropping out of doing and entering easily into a state of just being. It can be helpful to connect the breath to the process of dropping into inner listening. Take a big sigh. Prepare to rest into stillness however you are seated or lying.

1. Invite some of the settling prompts from Chapter 2 to arise naturally. Don't worry if the exact wording is different from usual, simply welcome whatever you can easily recall.

2. How about trying out some invitations for intuitive intention to arise? Simply read these words and notice how they land in the body: All that I am is welcome to be. All that I hear is welcome to be. All that I feel is welcome to be. Just as it is.

3. Invite an attitude of inner listening as you read these words and notice your embodied response to them: With great respect and love, I honor my heart, my inner teacher.

4. How about this one: I make inner harmony my first priority.

5. How about simply noticing: Just to be here is enough.

6. If you sense any of these three statements resonate a positive response in your body, perhaps repeat it again, and then use this phrase as you listen to the next recording of yoga nidrā, which gives you space and time to repeat an intention as you get to ingredient 3 in the recipe.

7. If none of the three intentions resonate with you, either return to the body sensing or invite whatever statement might feel more meaningful to you in this space.

8. Gently increase your breath volume and externalize your senses slowly, using the palming closure exercise from Chapter 2 to finish your practice.

Ways to inner listening #2 – Intention inquiry

If you are seeking direction or clarity, it may be more helpful to let your practice of yoga nidrā be guided by a particular intention. Instead of imposing a specific goal or desire upon the practice of yoga nidrā, how about inquiring, just asking questions? There is a big difference between asking questions directly, when you are fully conscious and alert, and asking the same questions when you are in the space of yoga nidrā.

Here is a way to invite intention to arise intuitively. Simply cycle through these questions as you read them and then listen to the same series of inquiries again in the space of yoga nidrā, after you have completed a settling process.

1. How does it feel just to be here in this effortless space of yoga nidrā?

2. If insight or intuitive guidance arises effortlessly, how can it be welcomed in most simply?

3. Encouraging gentle reminder: 'Now is the time simply to know that the whole of me is welcome to rest. To be here is more than enough.'

Watch the next breath and then continue.

1. If I were to frame an intention for this practice, I wonder, what would that be, and what would that intention feel like?

2. How about if I were to give myself permission to listen or to feel or sense the intuitive voice of my innermost guide, the guide that always honors and respects my highest and best interests; I wonder, what might I hear or feel?

3. Would this insight come in words, feelings, or sensations?

Ways to inner listening #3 – Embodied intuition

Often, because yoga nidrā is an embodied practice, with emphasis upon settling into physical comfort before all else, intuitive guidance can arise within the body. Here is a series of inquiries to encourage an embodied connection to intuition.

1. If I were to keep curious enough to welcome intuitive wisdom, where in the spaces inside the body would this wisdom rest right now?

2. Would I feel gut wisdom in my belly?

3. Perhaps the presence of wisdom is resting in the pelvis or the spine. And how's that?

4. How is this wisdom sensed or felt in these bones?

5. Or joints?

6. Or organs?

7. Perhaps this intuitive wisdom speaks most clearly from the heart.

8. Or maybe, I feel this wisdom in the throat.

9. Encouraging gentle reminder: The inherent intuitive wisdom of life itself resides in every cell of this resting body. This being is part of all of life.

Nidrista story: Being in grief with yoga nidrā

Yoli Maya Yeh Joseph, a Chicago educator working at the intersection of Indigenous preservation, healing, and social justice, facilitates community yoga nidrā grief circles. These yoga nidrā experiences intentionally hold space for grieving around race-based trauma, harm, and loss. Yoli explains, 'The cyclical nature of grief means that even though a clear intention is set, it is not possible to predict the response of participants. Some grieving folks find yoga nidrā to be a great solace and comfort, a respite from the hard and exhausting work of grieving. Others discover it deepens their sadness, and still others find yoga nidrā to be a valuable part of the long-term processing of individual and collective grief experiences, including ancestral grief. There is no right or wrong way to grieve. The yoga nidrā practice that feels very unhelpful today may turn out to be just what you need tomorrow.' It is important to choose a facilitator skilled in grief work if you intend to use yoga nidrā specifically to support grieving. Find out more about Yoli Maya Yeh's decolonizing grief and healing work in the resources section at the end of the book.

Now that we've explored the different ways you can choose to engage with intuition and intention, or simply welcome whatever arises, it's time to taste the next ingredient in every yoga nidrā recipe, the traveling of awareness around your resting body.

Chapter 4

Welcoming Attention
around the Body

Journeying through places and spaces

*remember that this tiredness
is a call from life itself
to return to yoga nidrā
so that every place can rest –
remember now this body here is nourished and renewed
by the act of doing nothing and receiving all it needs*

The fourth ingredient of yoga nidrā is a journey of attention through your resting body. Only the mental attention travels, while the body remains still. Often called a rotation of consciousness, the journey begins after the invitation for intuitive intention, and is usually followed by pairs of opposites.

There are innumerable itineraries across different schools of yoga nidrā, and in our teacher trainings, we share multiple approaches to encourage trainees to get familiar with a variety of routes. To make it easy to do yoga nidrā for yourself, we have chosen to focus attention on just one main itinerary in all the yoga nidrā recipes in this book. Each of the yoga nidrā recipes so far has used the same rotation of consciousness that moves from the crown of the head to the soles of the feet in a simple downward movement. We've deliberately repeated the same itinerary for this mental tour of the body in every recipe so that you can gain familiarity with the process. We have chosen the head-to-toes rotation of consciousness for three reasons:

1. It's easy to follow and easy to remember!

2. It's swift, efficient, and adaptable. It works well in a very short yoga nidrā and can be used to extend the practice by bringing more detail into specific parts, like face, hands, or feet. You don't need to learn a different itinerary for a short practice or a long practice because this one is so very versatile.

3. It's the most authentic original form of the rotation that we have been able to find.

You may remember that the earliest written references to yoga nidrā are found in ancient Indian praises to the many powers of the goddess, including the power of sleep: nidrā shakti. In these sources, carrying the attention on a journey around the physical body is so important that it's called the seed of the practice; the process of guiding awareness through the entire body is sometimes accompanied by gestures or sounds intended to protect the whole person by naming each part of the body in a specific sequence.

In modern yoga nidrā processes, movement of awareness is usually done without any sound or movement. You simply rest and carry your mental attention from one body part to the next, distributing energy and attention evenly.

Multiple journeys around the body

Journeys of awareness around the body are common to all yoga nidrā methods. Some routes begin in hands or feet, and some on face or head. They may use a variety of instruction or invitations to bring attention from one part to the next, but they all usually follow smooth paths connecting different parts of the body together. Many of the standard rotations privilege the right-hand side as the only acceptable starting point, and most exclude genitals, but we have discovered no good reason not to begin a rotation on the left-hand side, nor any sound rationale to exclude genitals if their inclusion supports the intention of the practice. No single route is correct: There is no right or wrong way around the body; it all depends on your intention for the practice.

▶ *Need to know*

Can I still practice yoga nidrā if I do not have both legs/ arms, or have less (or more) than the usual number of fingers/toes, or if I have had any organs removed?

Yes. It may support your practice if you adapt the rotation to suit your needs. Some people report a positive sense that movement of awareness around the body reaffirms the experience of wholeness, because at the level of vital energies, the body is always whole. All original organs, limbs, or other parts remain present in the energy body even if they are not physically present now. Others find that connecting to the named missing body part or organ can trigger phantom limb pain in that place. In the first case, the rotation of consciousness does not need to be altered, because it is possible to experience it in the energies of the body. In the second case, it makes more sense to adjust the standard rotations of consciousness to avoid mentioning the missing part or organ, or to choose some of the more spacious rotations that do not include so much detail.

Why is this ingredient included at this point in the process?

One of the main reasons for including the journey of attention in yoga nidrā is that it occupies the mind so completely that thoughts often tend to quieten down, so it becomes easier for us to rest. It also reconnects mental attention to our physicality, enhancing our capacity to feel embodied and present, accepting all sensations arising.

As mental awareness moves around the body, it activates a variety of locations in the motor and sensory cortices of the brain, and this can induce a sense of feeling very settled and whole. Some people also report that the rotation of consciousness can change their relationship to pain, reduce tremors, or generate feelings of warmth and well-being in every place. There is evidence that guiding mental attention around the body in this way can support recovery from brain injuries, including concussion, hemorrhage, and neural damage sustained after being struck by lightning.[17]

Your individual response to this ingredient of yoga nidrā depends largely on the way it is delivered. Some schools of yoga use a very bossy military tone in this part of the practice and keep a quick marching pace, while others are more spacious. We invite you simply to welcome the whole body with respect and kindness. The guidance that follows is composed of invitations and encouragements rather than instructions.

Nidrista story: Yoga nidrā rotation for pain relief

Jan experiences intense pain through osteoarthritis, a debilitating long-term illness that limits her mobility and makes it hard for her to sleep. She regularly uses a self-guided rotation through the night. 'I rarely get through the rotation all in one go. I often fall asleep and wake up in the tail end of a sleep cycle, then I remember where I had got to. Sometimes my journey around the body can take up to five hours or more. I rest the whole time. I feel such relief from pain and notice a massive improvement in the quality of my sleep when I practice yoga nidrā.'

Walking the same path with familiarity and ease

Every school of yoga nidrā has its own method of guiding this process. It can be interesting to explore the different journeys by listening to yoga nidrā practices from different schools, but to begin, we recommend sticking to the same rotation repeatedly, which is what we've done throughout this book. The easiest way to benefit from this ingredient of yoga nidrā is to become very familiar with just one itinerary of the journey around the body: Read through all the transcripts, listen to the audio tracks, make your own recordings, and then pick the one you like the best and maybe memorize the sequence.

Feeling your way round

To experience this journey of attention we recommend you first simply read it all the way through, feeling into each part of the body as you read. Then, when you listen to the recording it will be familiar, and your attention will flow easily. The ultimate intention is that, with practice, you won't need recordings or notes because you will intuitively embody this simple flow in your body. It might take a little time, but it will be worth it because then you will easily be able to do yoga nidrā by yourself anywhere, without the need for any external help from others' words.

The full journey of all 108 invitations takes about nine minutes, so set your timer. To get you started, there are two very easy, short versions of the same itinerary before the start of the full rotation. It is a good idea to read and listen to these first a few times before moving on to the complete journey. We've divided the journey into numbered sections, with body parts grouped together so that it is easier to follow.

Whether you are doing the complete tour or just the easy summaries, it is important to be settled and comfortable before you begin. This journey repeatedly invites you to sweep attention from left to right and then from right to left in a hypnotic rhythm. It can be deeply restful, so be sure to externalize your awareness fully as you exit the practice. Take a moment to recall the palming exit exercise from Chapter 2 to be sure you can get the most from these rotations.

▶ *Need to know*

I twitch/shudder/shake during yoga nidrā practice.
Is this normal?

Yes and no. Some small twitches are perfectly usual as the body settles into yoga nidrā. Sometimes bigger shudders arise or shaking occurs, and occasionally people experience waves of orgasmic release, especially during the rotation of consciousness. Usually, all these experiences pass through quite swiftly as excess energy is released, and then the body can settle into stillness again. With certain conditions such as restless legs, it can be helpful to press the soles of the feet into the floor or the wall to ground the movements. Sometimes, these twitches or shudders are unusually fierce or very disturbing, or they are related to a pre-existing health condition and simply manifest during yoga nidrā. Notice what arises for you with regular practice. If the shuddering or twitching increases in intensity or duration, it may be wise to check in with your facilitator and/or health-care providers to explore why this is happening for you.

Easy rhythmic journey of attention around the body #1

Rhythmic travels by numbers

You can follow this recipe by reading and directing attention around your body as you read, or if you prefer, you can listen to audio track 4.1 (see listing on page 1).

1. From crown of head

2. to scalp it flows,

3. from forehead

4. to these brows, the settling body now receives the nourishment of rest.

5. Between the brows,

6. through resting eyes,

7. the eyelids, right and left,

8. between the eyes, the rest is here, and all they see is welcomed in.

9. Within the ears,

10. behind the ears, these places now can rest.

11. The nostrils welcome every breath,

12. and both the lips

13. and tongue are nourished now by restfulness, are nurtured now by rest.

14. The teeth

15. and throat,

16. the uvula,

17. the arched roof of the mouth, are resting, settling into quiet, in yoga nidrā now.

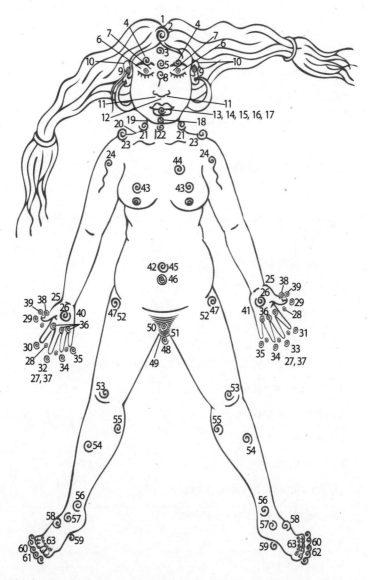

Rhythmic travels by numbers [Easy Journey #1. Audio track 4.1]

18. This chin is still because there is nothing to be said.

19. The back of neck,

20. the whole of spine,

21. and both sides of the neck,

22. the throat pipe now is soft within, all resting here and settling into yoga nidrā now.

23. Across the shoulders,

24. down both arms,

25. and into hands this flows. The yoga nidrā state is here to nourish and restore.

26. The palms of hands

27. and fingertips,

28. the spaces in between,

29. the thumbs

30. and index fingers of both hands are resting now.

31. On left and right,

32. from hand to hand,

33. the middle fingers

34. and the fourth,

35. both little fingers resting, too,

36. and all the webbing in between.

37. The fingertips

38. and cuticles,

39. the nails of both these hands,

40. on right and left,

41. on left and right, the whole of both hands now can rest. Every place is nurtured now by this.

42. Both palms and belly now can just be resting in this place. This yoga nidrā time is now, and every breath is rest.

43. From belly up to chest and breasts, there is a flow of restfulness.

44. Within this heart, a space to be attentive to the pulse, allows the heart and mind to be,

45. whilst stomach receives rest,

46. so centered in the navel is the nourishment of rest.

47. Both hips and

48. genitals can rest,

49. anus and

50. pelvis, too,

51. whilst all throughout the pelvic floor, this rest is nurturing.

52. These hips

53. and knees,

54. these shanks

55. and calves,

56. the ankles

57. and both feet, are welcomed in the resting place of yoga nidrā now.

58. The tops of feet,

59. the soles

60. and toes,

61. the right foot

62. and the left,

63. the spaces in between the toes are settled into rest.

No need to take another step, the place to be is here.

Easy journey of attention around the body #2

Nine encouraging reminders to embody the experience of yoga nidrā

You can follow this recipe by reading and directing attention around your body as you read, or if you prefer, you can listen to audio track 4.2 (see listing on page 1).

1. I know I am welcome to rest now.

2. The nourishment of rest is welcomed as a guest into this body.

3. The home of this body makes a welcome for rest.

4. Every place in this body receives rest in every space.

5. The nourishment of rest is arriving now along the front of this body.

6. I welcome rest in the back of this body.

7. Rest nurtures the left side of this body.

8. Rest nourishes the right side of this body.

9. I welcome rest into the whole of this body.

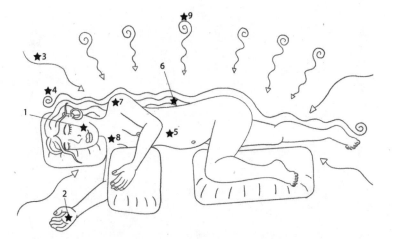

Nine encouraging reminders to embody yoga nidrā
[Easy Journey #2. Audio track 4.2]

Easy journey of attention around the body #3

Complete tour (108 invitations)

This is a longer process, and after a while, your attention will flow effortlessly around the whole body in this way. But do be patient as it might take time to feel confident with the complete tour. Following are our top helpful memory tips.

First, simply listen to an audio of the complete tour. The best thing is to record your own. If you prefer, to get started, you can listen to audio track 4.3 (see listing on page 1). Listen a few times, and then use the illustration below to help you track the different places. It is helpful to take it slowly, focusing on the groups of body parts in each place.

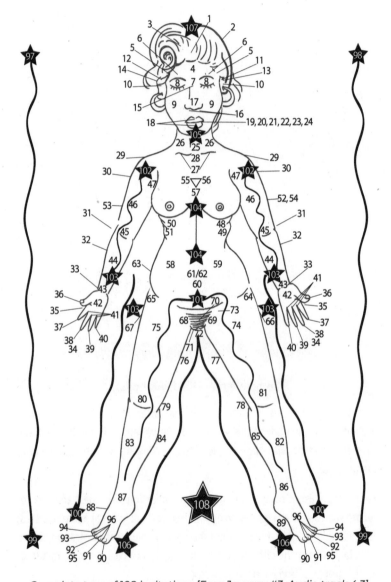

Complete tour of 108 invitations [Easy Journey #3. Audio track 4.3]

You can also make your own drawing and follow around the whole tour with your pencil or finger while listening to the audio. Then return to just listening to the audio. After a few repetitions, it rapidly gets easier and easier to remember the process effortlessly. In the end, it doesn't feel like you are having to 'remember' anything, it simply happens by itself. A key tip is simply to recall that the tour is always flowing downward, and that you cannot get this wrong, because this is your practice!

Be sure to ask of every place: How is the nourishment of rest being welcomed here now? How about this place? Please be aware that these invitations group the individual parts together to make it easier to flow the attention around the body.

Inviting rest to nourish this body: head and face

1. crown of head
2. back of head
3. whole of scalp, all the way through
4. whole of forehead
5. both temples, left and right
6. both eyebrows, right and left
7. space between eyebrows
8. left eye and right eye, right eyelid and left
9. cheeks, left and right
10. ears, right and left
11. spaces inside left ear
12. spaces inside right ear
13. behind right ear

14. behind left ear
15. center of head

Inviting rest to nourish this body: nose, mouth, and jaw

16. inside left nostril, inside right nostril
17. tip of nose, and whole of nose
18. upper lip and lower lip, meeting place between the lips
19. upper gums and lower gums
20. front teeth, back teeth
21. space between upper and lower teeth
22. floor of mouth, roof of mouth
23. inside of cheeks, right and left
24. jaws and tongue

Inviting rest to nourish this body: neck, shoulders, and arms

25. front of throat and back of neck
26. left side of neck, and right
27. collarbones, right and left
28. space between collarbones
29. tops of shoulders, left and right
30. along outer sides of upper arms, right and left
31. tips of elbows, left and right
32. outer sides of forearms, right and left
33. backs of wrists, left and right

Inviting rest to nourish this body: both hands, fingers, and thumbs

34. tips of all fingers and tips of both thumbs, left hand and right

35. spaces in between all the fingers, on right hand and left

36. both thumbs, left and right, tips and base

37. both index fingers, tips and base, right and left

38. both middle fingers, tips and base, left and right

39. fourth fingers on both hands, tips and base, right and left

40. two little fingers, tips and base, left and right

41. webbing in between all the fingers

Inviting rest to nourish this body: back up the arms

42. palms of both hands, right and left

43. inner wrists, left and right

44. inner forearms, right and left

45. inner elbows, left and right

46. inner surface of upper arms, right and left

47. armpits, left and right

Inviting rest to nourish this body: chest, front and back

48. left ribs

49. spaces between left ribs

50. right ribs

51. spaces between right ribs

52. left shoulder blade

53. right shoulder blade

54. space between two shoulder blades
55. front of breastbone
56. behind front of breastbone
57. center of chest, betwixt breastbone and space between two shoulder blades

Inviting rest to nourish this body: belly and pelvis

58. right side of belly
59. left side of belly
60. whole of the belly
61. navel
62. spine behind belly
63. lower back
64. left hip
65. right hip

Inviting rest to nourish this body: buttocks and groins

66. right buttock
67. left buttock
68. right groin
69. left groin
70. pubic bones
71. tail bone
72. floor of pelvis
73. whole of pelvis

Inviting rest to nourish this body: legs

74. top of left thigh
75. top of right thigh
76. back of right thigh
77. back of left thigh
78. back of left knee
79. back of right knee
80. top of right knee
81. top of left knee
82. left shin
83. right shin
84. right calf
85. left calf

Inviting rest to nourish this body: feet and toes

86. left ankle
87. right ankle
88. top of right foot
89. sole of left foot
90. big toes, right and left
91. both second toes, left and right
92. both third toes, right and left
93. both fourth toes, left and right
94. both little toes, right and left
95. tips of all the toes
96. all spaces in between the toes on both feet

Inviting rest to nourish this body: main body parts

(Encouraging reminder: whole body all together)

97. whole right side of this body is nourished by rest

98. whole left side of this body is nourished by rest

99. both sides of this body together are nourished by rest

100. left leg and right leg are nourished by rest

101. legs and pelvis are nourished by rest

102. right arm and left arm are nourished by rest, both arms together are nourished by rest

103. all the limbs are nourished by rest

104. chest and belly are nourished by rest

105. head, neck, and spine are nourished by rest

106. tips of toes to crown of head,

107. scalp to skin on soles of feet:

108. the whole of this body is nourished by rest

End of the journey around the body.

Be sure to take the time to come around, slowly externalizing your awareness before moving.

As you've experienced in the previous yoga nidrā recipes, the completion of the tour of awareness around the body is usually followed by pairs of opposites, and this is the main ingredient of the next chapter.

Chapter 5

Playing with Paradox and Integration

Inviting pairs of opposites

*yoga nidrā – this is nothing – this is everything I feel
beneath all daily actions that this body moves through here
is a rhythmic pulse of lifetimes resting softly in the heart –
from periphery to center in this place where I come home
is a yoga nidrā welcome to a space of balance here*

*in the middle of all chaos
at circumference of this strife
is a breath between the tears and a sweet joy between the griefs
at the threshold of this turning breath
a stillness can be found*

Paradox is right at the heart of yoga nidrā. When you practice yoga nidrā, you may look like you are just taking a nap, but in your rest, you are fully awakened to your true nature. *Awakened Sleep* was the title of the first book on yoga nidrā ever published in Europe,[18] and the sense of resting awakened within sleep encapsulates the essential nature of yoga nidrā.

By this stage, having experienced a few different yoga nidrā recipes, you are probably beginning to wake up to the fact that this deeply restful process can be profoundly rejuvenating; you may seem dead to the outside world, but when you practice yoga nidrā, you can be wide awake to your inner world of potential, healing, and creativity. At the beginning of the book, we introduced the idea of yoga nidrā as an experience of paradox, a place in which we could be awake and asleep at the same time, and this chapter sets out just how important this idea is in practical terms.

Pairs of opposites are essential ingredients in all forms of yoga nidrā. Usually, they are explicitly named and placed after the journey of attention around the body. Occasionally, the pairing of opposites is implicit, such as sensing how the individual places we have noticed in the body rotation exist in relation to each other; but more often, this section of the practice invites us to create deliberately contrasting images or experiences.

Frequently, the pairs of opposites in yoga nidrā present opportunities to imagine two different sensations, for example evoking the sense of being heavy and then being light, or being huge and then tiny.

In some yoga nidrā schools there can be an invitation to explore opposite emotions, such as sadness and joy, or anger and contentment. It is common to be instructed

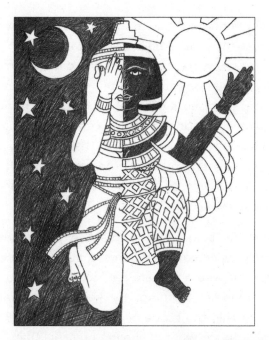

*Simple pairs of opposites such as 'night and day'
provide cues to observe contrasting sensations and
experiences, first separately and then together.*

to alternate between the two opposite experiences,
feeling first one and then the other, and then repeating
the contrast. Often at this stage in yoga nidrā, we may be
invited to bring the pair of contrasting sensations or feelings
together, to hold the possibility that the two very different
experiences we just imagined currently coexist, or that we
can be a witness to the presence of them both together.

It is not always easy to conjure up emotions or sensations
when instructed to do so, even in the state of yoga nidrā.

Some people find it tricky to imagine feeling hot or cold just because the yoga nidrā instructor tells them to. It is not always easy to alternate between two different imagined states if you are not entirely certain about how each one feels in the first place. It can make it hard to continue with the practice if you don't want to cultivate the particular emotion named by the facilitator at that moment, or if you cannot actually remember a time when you felt deeply happy, or very warm, or whatever it is that you are being instructed to evoke.

To make this stage of the practice easier, we have deliberately selected ingredients that are immediately obvious, right where you are resting, so that you do not have to imagine anything. By keeping the range of opposites within the scope of current experience, all you need do is notice what is already present. That is easier than trying to imagine things that may not seem very real or accessible to you.

▶ *Need to know*

I can hear my belly making lots of noise during yoga nidrā. Is this normal?

This is a very good sign indeed! It's an indication your body is relaxing. If your gut is gurgling, it is probably because your practice of yoga nidrā is permitting available energy and circulation to be directed to support the digestive process, or to alert you to the fact that you are ready for your next meal. It's a parasympathetic response of the nervous system, permitting rest and repair. It could be sounds of the digestive system or the lymphatic system. Either way, it's good news.

Observable paradox in the here and now

During yoga nidrā, there is no shortage of opposites readily observable in the body and immediate environment. Even the process of settling down in the first five minutes offers a vast selection of opposites from which to choose, including:

❖ recent shift from vertical to horizontal

❖ process of settling from movement into stillness

❖ contrast between having been active and now resting

❖ continued activities outside while you rest still on your mat

❖ hearing sounds very close to you and those very far away

❖ sensing breath coming in and going out

❖ observing the surface beneath you and the space above

❖ feeling front of body and back

❖ being aware of right side of body and left

When these very simple opposites are presented, almost everybody can connect with them quite easily and often start noticing opposites of their own without any effort.

Once the opposites can be sensed, people can continue with the process of yoga nidrā without struggling to imagine or remember whatever they are told, because all they have to do is notice what is happening right now.

This is a radical simplification of the process of yoga nidrā. It takes the process out of the facilitator's control and puts it in the hands of the practitioner (that's you!), who is then far more likely to be able to practice by themselves. Our intention is to support your own practice of yoga nidrā, so we offer you elements that are naturally arising and easy to notice.

Why is this ingredient included at this point in the process?

Pairs of opposites are potent in the yoga nidrā mix. We create powerful energy when we bring together two strongly contrasting experiences. In our minds, it is simply not possible to hold a pair of opposites together because we cannot feel two totally different things at the precise same time. Even in the extraordinary and delightful experience of what looks like laughing and crying at the same time, we are in fact rapidly switching between these two states.

When, in the restful process of yoga nidrā, we invite the mind to play the game of noticing two contrasting experiences simultaneously, we tend to abandon logic and leap with freedom into a more intuitive space, which is why yoga nidrā can be such a boost for energy and creativity. Sometimes, we just give up the struggle and rest somewhere outside of the two opposites, which can be profoundly nourishing too. Either way, playing with paradox in this way can liberate us from the limits of logical and cognitive thought. It frees the imagination.

Freedom from attachment to either one of the contrasting pair of opposites can help us cultivate balance. A positive outcome of practicing pairs of opposites in yoga nidrā is that we start to spot them turning up in everyday life. Then the capacity we have cultivated in yoga nidrā, to observe the two opposites together, becomes a very valuable life skill, as we navigate with greater awareness the seesaw of human experiences, between moments of deep grief and elation, or times of struggle and ease.

Practicing playing with paradox

To practice these pairs of opposites, we recommend you first read the whole list, feeling into each invitation as you read. Then when you listen to the recording, the invitations will be familiar, and you'll more easily be able to follow the suggestions.

Once you've read and listened a few times, you may find that you can recall the sequence of opposites easily. In the end, you won't need the recording or the words, and you won't even need to try and remember the opposites presented in this book. You can just feel confident to welcome whatever opposites arise naturally and intuitively in response to your surroundings and what is happening in your life. With a small amount of practice, you will easily be able to welcome whatever opposites arise when you settle down to practice, and notice them in your life without following a script.

The complete set of suggestions for opposites takes about five to 10 minutes.

Set your timer to call you back – it's easy to get lost in the heart of the labyrinth.

To get you started, there is a very easy, short version to try first. Whether you are doing the long or short versions, be sure to precede them with your choice of settling processes. Finish up with an externalizing process from Chapter 2. If you like, to get started, you can listen to audio track 5.0 (see listing on page 2).

Easy opposites recipe #1

1. Encouraging reminder: All these parts are resting now. And the whole of this body is resting.

2. How would it be to welcome the parts and the whole to rest together at the same time? And now, right now, are there parts of this resting body that are sleeping?

3. And is this mind perhaps alert and attentive, perhaps watching the body sleep?

4. How about being aware of being asleep or awake, alert or resting?

5. Or both together?

6. How would it feel to be alert and resting at the same time?

7. How would it feel to be asleep and awake at the same time?

8. How about being alert and restful at the same time, simultaneously awake and sleeping?

Easy (rhythmic) opposites recipe #2

This recipe incorporates the opposites in the rhythmic yoga nidrā at the end of the introduction (page 26), so flip back to there, skip straight to the 'settling in' section (step 2), and bookmark it.

Take a moment, even as you rest here now, to exhale and inquire into these preparatory pairs of opposites:

Even if there's chaos in my life, and/or mind, and/or feelings and/ or world, am I able to give myself the time to stop for this now?

However and whatever I am feeling in this moment, how about I just let myself be, just as I am?

Now return to the place you have bookmarked, and reread through to the end of the 'playing with paradox' section (step 5). Feel into the pairs of opposites as you rest, and then skip to the externalizing and completion sections (steps 8 and 9).

Chapter 6

Optional Connecting to Imaginative Capacity

Feeling into sensory and extrasensory knowing, for inspiration, healing, and nurturing

this receptive place of nidrā
gifts us time to heal and feel
how long-dormant inspiration may awaken as we rest –
reclaiming creativity by resting in the space
where patient answers quietly wait for rediscovery

Of all the ingredients in the nidrā recipes, this is the one that we most often leave out. The restorative experience of yoga nidrā is perfectly effective without this section, so if welcoming connection to the imaginative faculty doesn't appeal to you, we simply invite you to skip it.

This part of the cycle usually comes after the pairs of opposites and before savoring the second intuitive intention. Often, many people have by now moved into a trance of such profound stillness that their senses are fully turned to the interior world. In this place, practitioners may not consciously hear all or any instructions that are delivered by an external voice. If the hearing faculty is still operational, then this can be a receptive time to welcome connection to imagination, memory, and inspiration. Any guidance or invitations that are provided or surface naturally may be welcomed very deeply within.

Seeing things?

This sixth ingredient in the yoga nidrā recipe is most often called visualization. This is not a very helpful term, because so many people find it hard to visualize, especially if they are being told what they are supposed to be seeing, and it doesn't appear. It is much easier and more useful to think of this as an invitation to connect with imaginative capacity through whatever sensory or extrasensory means is most vivid for you. In our list of ingredients, we prefer to refer to this part of the practice as '*optional* connecting to imaginative capacity – feeling into sensory and extrasensory knowing.'

In traditional forms of yoga nidrā, at this point in the practice people are usually instructed to look into the mind's eye, or the space where dreams appear at night, and to 'see' there whatever the instructor tells them to see. Often, rapid individual images or archetypal symbols are described. Sometimes, the facilitator will outline a scenario or tell a story in which the practitioner can see themselves as a participant. Occasionally, instructors convey information or unfold complex narratives in this section of the yoga nidrā. The direction (and it is mostly an order) is usually to imagine that the described images are being projected like a movie on the inside of the participant's forehead, or behind the inside of the closed eyelids, in a space referred to as the 'mind sky' (*chidakash* in Sanskrit).

All these images are effectively imposed by the instructor on the imagination of the practitioner. They are not always easy to follow, and they often cause confusion or concern in people who might feel that they are 'not getting it.' Sometimes the images are beneficial, welcome, and enjoyable, and sometimes they are not. It's unpredictable. Previous trauma can be inadvertently triggered by well-intentioned facilitators who do not quite realize what reactions may be provoked by the images they are offering. The trouble arises when triggering images pop up without any warning, coming as a bit of a surprise in the middle of a relaxing nidrā.

The enormous benefit of doing your own yoga nidrā practice is that the images in your recipe will not be impositions from an external voice, but instead will arise from within yourself. This is a good incentive for learning to cook your own yoga nidrā recipes so that you can use this ingredient for inspiration, healing, and nurture.

▶ Need to know

I can't visualize at all, can I still practice yoga nidrā?

Yes. It is not necessary to visualize during yoga nidrā. A complete and effective practice of nidrā does not depend upon the visualization of images, but is founded upon the capacity to rest and observe and notice bodily sensation with attentive interest.

Many people are unable to visualize, but do find it easy to recognize sensory input such as sounds, smells, or touch. There is absolutely no need to be able to conjure up visual images in yoga nidrā. Many people report that if they are instructed to imagine specific images, they completely blank, but when invited to witness sensations, or to respond to more general prompts, then they can envision vividly. The invitation 'Maybe you find yourself in a delightful garden with flowers blooming?' tends to get a better response than a demand to 'See the red rose.' If we remain curious and receptive at this time, then many vivid and often unexpected images can appear unbidden in the mind's eye. This is the part of the cyclical process of nidrā where we may also receive embodied signs or prompts for actions to take in the waking state.

Why is this ingredient included at this point in the process?

The main reason this is included in many yoga nidrā methods is to cultivate imaginative capacity. It is more nourishing for the imagination to invite your own images to arise than it is to have them prescribed for you. Some facilitators also utilize this section to impart esoteric teachings, to facilitate ancestral connections, or remember dreams – and this is certainly a receptive space to foster such connections. At a more practical level, this section of the nidrā is an excellent moment to do some problem-solving, because it is fertile ground for harvesting creative solutions (see Chapter 13).

Nidrista story: Overcoming fear of flying

'It all started with landing in a storm,' explains Pawel, a Polish yoga therapist, who clocked up thousands of air miles, flying around Europe to deliver trainings. 'My heart would race, and I'd get cold sweats. My body would contract and shiver each time the plane was up in the sky. Every trip was a traumatic experience. I was unable to walk, eat anything, or even go to the bathroom. I would be so ill by the time I arrived that it would take two days to recover. The fear was overwhelming. I was not afraid of take-off or landing, but of being up there.' Pawel spent years trying to solve his problem logically. He met with pilots and first officers, cabin crew, and air traffic controllers. He even studied aerodynamics so he could understand logically just how safe the planes were. 'But the more I learned, the worse the fear got: Intellectually, I knew I didn't need to be frightened, but I was still totally unable to control my body.'

Eventually Pawel and Nirlipta used the process of yoga nidrā to help Pawel embody, in the sixth stage of the practice, a sensory and fully somatic knowing that he could trust himself to feel safe in planes. They were not classic visualizations of images, but more of a process of physically embodying the experience of trusting that the plane was a safe place to be. 'This therapeutic application of yoga nidrā had an immediate effect on the physiological effects of my fear. One week after the session, I had a delightful flight. I was not only able to walk but also to spend the time of the flight effectively – writing articles, preparing for the trainings, and practicing yoga nidrā.' Pawel used journaling to deepen and consolidate his new confidence in flying. The following is part of a poem he wrote to explain how yoga nidrā had helped free him from this debilitating phobia.

> *By the power of sleep*
> *I learn to see*
> *the streams of habits*
> *I used to think I am.*

We recommend keeping your approach to this ingredient simple, open, and curious. Don't rush. Take your time to feel your way into what works easily for you here. Instead of instructing yourself to see images in the mind's eye, we encourage you to welcome whatever sensory or extrasensory form of connection that may surface from your imaginative capacity. You may not 'see,' but you may feel the connections you are inviting as an embodied sensation, or they may come in the form of inner voices, or the wordless song of your own knowing. However they surface, this is a place to feel confident that there is no way you can do this wrong because this is *your* practice of yoga nidrā, and if you don't like what arises, you can leave it aside and move on to the next ingredient.

▶ *Need to know*

I'm recovering from or preparing for surgery. Is it safe to practice yoga nidrā?

Yes. Yoga nidrā can be very supportive for recovery after surgical operations. Many people report that listening to back-to-back nidrā helps manage pain immediately after surgery, and others have found that practicing during convalescence, especially using positive visualizations or other sensory invitations for wellness, can support healing. It can also be an effective way to relieve anxiety prior to surgery.

Although it is not a necessary part of yoga nidrā, ingredient 6 can be a very valuable, enjoyable aspect of the practice. Here are nine nourishing serving suggestions to enrich your experience with this optional element of the process.

Nine serving suggestions to connect to imaginative capacity

You can simply make the following connections in any yoga nidrā of your choice that includes space and time to taste these different serving suggestions.

❖ Do nothing. Simply feel or watch what happens.

> Next time you get to this stage of yoga nidrā, just pause, and know that it is more than enough simply to be here. Just rest. This may not seem like the most creative use of your time, but being in this place, without expectation or anticipation, can be immensely nurturing and nourishing, and in the end, far more rewarding.

❖ Take a stroll in your imagination.

> You can go anywhere you like. Visit your favorite places and soak up the good memories, or visit imaginary lands, locations from movies, or sacred landscapes.

❖ Invite in colors and light.

> Fill your mind's eye or your interior world with favorite shades and hues, or paint a rainbow in the mind sky. Staying curious and welcoming, you may find yourself inhabiting exquisite dream colorscapes.

❖ Visit a friend.

> Living or dead, old, or new – enjoy tea and conversation with your favorite people.

❖ Hear music.

> Listen into the mind's ear, chill to heavenly vibes, or enjoy a concert by your favorite band.

❖ Invite in a dream scenario.

> If there is a dream you would like to recall, bring a small fragment of the dream into this space of the nidrā and see if you can track its scent to retrieve the rest of it.

❖ Ask a question.

> Keep it simple. 'What's the next step?' or 'What happens now?' are helpful inquiries that can solicit good answers. Perhaps bring a particular issue into this nidrā space and see what happens.

❖ Meditate or pray.

> Use this time to do spiritual practice.

❖ Commune with the ancestors.

> Give thanks and praise to those upon whose shoulders you stand; remember you are your ancestors' wildest dreams! Invite their protection. They want to help.

For more recipes to boost creativity, see Chapter 13.

Overlaps and parallels

You may find that this part of the yoga nidrā recipe reminds you of dreams or of techniques you have previously encountered. Many people observe, when they first start to do yoga nidrā, that how they feel at this point in the practice reminds them of previous experiences they may have had in meditation, dreams, or trances. Images from these previous encounters with your dream life can sometimes show up when you arrive in this part of the yoga nidrā.

It is helpful to understand a little more about some of the many overlaps and parallels between yoga nidrā and other processes that use imaginative capacity, such as dreaming and meditation, so following, we've answered a few of the most frequently asked questions on these topics.

1. Am I dreaming in the visualization section of yoga nidrā?

    Maybe, maybe not. Most practices of yoga nidrā guide practitioners to states of restful awareness that are not specifically intended to lead into dreaming. Many people report that, during yoga nidrā, they drop in and out of fully awake alertness and deep unconscious sleep or navigate the threshold between those experiences. Some people observe that they drift easily from these threshold spaces into dreaming states, and may recall dreams, or flashes of dream memories – especially during this sixth section of yoga nidrā. All these experiences are possible, and so also is the experience of being lucidly aware of the distinct differences and the overlaps between these different experiences.

2. What's the difference between lucid dreaming and the visualization section in yoga nidrā?

    A lucid dream is one where we are consciously and cognitively aware of the fact that we are dreaming while we are dreaming. Yoga nidrā cultivates conscious familiarity with the experiences of falling asleep, teaching us to rest in the boundary places between sleep and dream with relaxed alertness. This is different from lucidity in dream. Lucid dreaming and yoga nidrā are two different experiences that can support each other.

Because it is possible sometimes to drift into a daydreaming trance while still awake in yoga nidrā, especially in section 6, the practice can become a direct interface between relaxed awareness of the onset of sleep and lucid dreaming. Whether or not this happens, yoga nidrā provides access to conscious experiences of the thresholds of waking and sleeping and tends to cultivate the capacity for dream recall; all these experiences can helpfully prepare for lucidity in dream.

3. What's the difference between the visualization section in yoga nidrā and meditation?

Some meditative practices use creative visualizations to invoke images of deities or light, and these can also appear in the sixth section of yoga nidrā. The key distinction is that in yoga nidrā we release all effort and stop 'doing.' Ultimately, of course, that can also be the intention in some meditative practices.

Yoga nidrā can be understood to be the meditative heart of yoga: by releasing any effort to be or to think, the practice invites us to drop into a state of simply being that is right at the heart of all yoga, including meditative practice. The difference between experiences of yoga nidrā and classic meditation practices is not just the fact that the meditation practice is vertical and yoga nidrā is usually horizontal.

The experience of visualization or meditative attention in yoga nidrā can feel more embodied than in many seated meditation methods. This is partly because the cyclical process of yoga nidrā involves many ingredients that directly engage with bodily perception, such as deeply relaxed settling, rotations of awareness, and pairs of opposites. These techniques require a level of embodied presence that may not typically be part of meditation practice.

There are so many different approaches to meditation that it is hard to generalize, but the boundaries between yoga nidrā and meditation can get very fuzzy, especially in this ingredient, and especially if we sometimes choose to practice yoga nidrā sitting, which is an option.

It's also possible to blur the distinctions between meditation and yoga nidrā even further by including meditative techniques within the structure of yoga nidrā. Mentally reciting mantras, focusing attention upon an internal version of a mandala, or even witnessing your resting self in yoga nidrā, doing a loving kindness meditation, are all options here.

There are also overlaps and parallels with hypnosis, which are explored in Chapter 7.

Nidrista story: Visions of the elixir of life

Brigid was undergoing an intensive program of chemotherapy to treat inflammatory breast cancer. She was very anxious and fearful and wanted to listen to a yoga nidrā practice while she received treatments. Working together with Uma in a series of one-to-one sessions, Brigid co-created her own special yoga nidrā for this challenging time. Co-creative yoga nidrā is a collaborative process between client and facilitator to integrate client visions and preferences within the yoga nidrā process, crafting unique yoga nidrā experiences for specific purposes.

In her chemotherapy nidrā, Brigid requested a visualization of what she described as the 'elixir or life,' not only for ingredient 6, but also for the rotation of consciousness. 'I want yoga nidrā to help me welcome chemotherapy and transform it into liquid golden light, the elixir of life. I want to feel it flowing like rivers and streams inside me,' she explained. 'I want to radiate that luminous golden fluid and share the elixir of life and pure love with everyone and everything on the planet.' Her vivid vision was incorporated into the fourth and sixth ingredients of her special yoga nidrā recipe so that the rotation of consciousness spread liquid golden light throughout every part of the body. When she arrived in section 8, Brigid would visualize herself radiating the healing qualities of this light, not just to benefit herself, but every living being on earth. Uma recorded a 20-minute nidrā with these ingredients, and Brigid listened to it every time she went to the hospital for chemo. 'It helped me to transform my fear into love,' she says.

Here are two serving suggestions for ingredient 6.

Serving suggestion #1

Encouraging intuition in a voice that you can trust

First, read through the following nine invitations and suggestions, and then record them in your own voice, or listen to audio track 6.0 (see listing page 2).

Take time to settle yourself, and cycle through your favorite versions of yoga nidrā ingredients 1 to 5.

Encourage yourself: 'Know that it is more than enough simply to be here and now, to be resting.'

Ask yourself a few questions.

How about…

1. just seeing myself resting here and now?

2. just seeing, in this mind's eye, myself now, breathing here?

3. watching myself resting here, from this moment now, right back through to the moment when I first lay down?

4. watching this body resting and breathing, from the very start of the practice up until right now and right here?

5. simply, kindly sensing myself for the whole time that I've been here, for the past 20 minutes?

6. just feeling this body here, in this place now, resting on just one small part of the whole world, one little place on the whole of the surface of the earth?

7. simply sensing the huge size of this planet earth, and at the same time seeing this little place where I rest, as just one tiny part of it?

8. just breathing in this place, sensing this tiny human form resting upon the vast surface of the planet earth, just resting in this moment?

9. letting go of this little game and knowing it is more than enough simply to be here and now, to be resting.

Serving suggestion #2

Seeing or sensing yourself in yoga nidrā

Repetition helps us consolidate confidence in self-guiding our own yoga nidrā. This serving suggestion returns to the nine-minute nidrā song at the end of the introduction. It is based on a classic yoga nidrā technique: the experience of 'seeing your own body' resting in nidrā, as if you could simply look down upon yourself with your mind's eye to watch yourself resting.

If you cannot literally 'see' yourself, then simply feel into the meeting places between your body and the floor beneath. You can try this one right now, just as you sit and read, and then welcome it into the process of your next yoga nidrā practice when you reach the sixth ingredient.

Flip back to page 26 and skip straight to the sixth step in the easy rhythmic nidrā, settle into the felt sense of the words, and keep a kindly eye on yourself as you read. Or feel free to listen to audio track 6.0 (see listing page 2).

In the next chapter, we move on to savor the intention that we first tasted with ingredient 3.

Returning to Inner Listening

*Savoring the flavor of your
yoga nidrā now*

*welcomed deep within our state of yoga nidrā here
we receive embodied wisdoms
these are intuition's gifts –
silent language
of this hidden inner voice is heard
within our rest –
we savor now
the taste of our intentions made before*

This chapter explores how to savor the intention planted in the third ingredient of yoga nidrā. Because yoga nidrā is a naturally cyclical process, we circle back to the start before we end, returning to the invitation for intuitive intention which we placed at the beginning. We are not the same as when we began, so when we revisit ingredient 3, it becomes ingredient 7. Although the two elements might carry the same name and address the same issue, they have different functions in the recipe of yoga nidrā. The easiest way to sense the difference between the two is to keep curious.

Because yoga nidrā is an effortless practice, sometimes there is no need to set a goal or a specific intention. Sometimes it is more appropriate simply to be in a space of listening curiously and welcoming whatever arises. It's as if the first intention (ingredient 3) is planting a seed, and the revisiting of this intention is gently checking to see how it has grown. You can choose to plant a certain kind of seed if you want to grow a certain kind of plant, or you can just be open to the idea of seeing what might grow by itself if you leave the earth be.

Whether or not you made a conscious choice about the third ingredient, the cyclical process of yoga nidrā will bring you into a different state by the time you reach the seventh ingredient, so you may receive some surprises when you return to see how the seed has grown. Alternatively, you may know for sure that you want to nourish the particular seed that you deliberately planted. In either case, curiosity is the wisest approach. You don't want to shut down the power of your unconscious mind to deliver some surprising outcomes. The following two examples give you a sense of what can happen at this point in the nidrā practice if you just remain curious.

Nidrista story: Effortlessly losing a bad habit without any intention

Mel was a lifelong nail-biter. She had bitten her nails for 54 years. It was so much part of who she thought she was that she did not even think of it as a bad habit. When she started practicing yoga nidrā daily as part of a training course with Nirlipta, Mel did not set any intention at all. She just enjoyed yoga nidrā and was curious to see what might happen if she did it every day. After four weeks, she had to buy a pair of nail clippers. 'One day, I simply noticed that I had long fingernails. They needed clipping for the first time in my life. And then I realized I wasn't a nail-biter anymore. My bad habit had simply disappeared. I no longer experienced any desire to bite my fingernails. I had made no conscious effort to break the habit; I made no resolutions about not biting my nails; I had just been practicing yoga nidrā and feeling more relaxed. I effortlessly lost the habit. Having to buy that pair of nail clippers was, for me, powerful evidence of the transformative power of yoga nidrā.'

Mel's experience is common, and her habit was a minor irritation. Other people have experienced the same process of effortless freedom from habits that can damage health and limit life, including serious addictions to nicotine and marijuana. Along the spectrum from a tendency to a habit, to an addiction, yoga nidrā can be a powerful ally.[19]

Nidrista story: Finding an egg in the nest – the power of curious intention

Adam, a software developer in his late twenties, had never even heard of yoga nidrā when he showed up for a session that Uma was teaching at a festival. He was super skeptical. Before he started, he proclaimed himself to be a 'total nonvisualizer.' 'I never, ever visualize things: When people describe images, colors, or objects, I simply cannot see anything. It just doesn't happen for me.' Adam did a 20-minute yoga nidrā practice. In it, people were invited to feel their physical body as a tree and to move awareness around the body as if around the branches, roots, and trunk of a tree. Ingredient 3 was an option to place a nest in the tree/body. This was the first invitation to taste the intention. Ingredient 7 was an option to revisit the nest, perhaps to look inside and see what was there. To his total delight and astonishment, Adam, the total nonvisualizer, clearly 'saw' a small sky-blue egg in his nest. More than that: 'I knew that the egg had a message for me, so I opened it. Inside was a tiny roll of paper. When I read the message written on it, it was the perfect answer to this massive IT problem I'd been working on for months. It was a brilliant solution, and I saw it. Nothing like this had ever happened to me before. I was completely thrilled and amazed.'

Neither Mel nor Adam set clear intentions for their practice. They both simply remained curious. Their unconscious mind, having their best interests at heart, was free to come up with helpful solutions to problems they had not even articulated consciously.

Yoga nidrā, trance, and hypnosis

The experience of yoga nidrā brings us into natural trance space, where the unconscious mind can provide simple and surprising solutions, as Mel and Adam discovered. Yoga nidrā is a form of yogic self-hypnosis, and many of the elements of the practice are also used in hypnotherapy. In clinical hypnosis, yoga nidrā ingredient 7 is described as a posthypnotic suggestion, and it is a powerful force for change, as you may discover for yourself.

▶ *Need to know*

Is yoga nidrā hypnosis?

Hypnotic phenomena arise in yoga nidrā because self-hypnosis techniques are incorporated into the basic process of the practice. The rotation of consciousness and the pairs of opposites both induce and deepen hypnotic trance, and the intention can be posthypnotic suggestion. Because these hypnotic ingredients are woven into the fabric of yoga nidrā, they can become familiar. As we practice, we learn how to guide ourselves through different states of trance with awareness. Ultimately, with practice, yoga nidrā becomes a method of conscious yogic self-hypnosis.

Nidrista story: Being in recovery – Yoga nidrā for addictions

Collette Caroll is a yoga nidrā facilitator in long-term recovery from chronic alcoholism through the Alcoholics Anonymous 12-step program. She leads yoga nidrā meditations to support other addicts. 'When I found yoga nidrā, I was already a yoga teacher with 10 years' sobriety. During my first practice of yoga nidrā at the Amrit Yoga Institute, I recognized immediately how helpful yoga nidrā can be for people in recovery. I came home from my yoga nidrā training and instantly began teaching for my friends in recovery. They, too, realized what I had experienced. We discovered together how yoga nidrā could dissolve the stigma and shame, the denial, resistance, physical compulsions, and mental obsessions of addiction. I simplified the practice, changing the words, and reorganized each component to ease the challenges of addiction and recovery. We need yoga nidrā invitations, not directives; we need welcoming to allow us to participate the way we choose.'

Learn more about yoga nidrā for recovery from addiction in the resources section at the end of the book.

Other ingredients of yoga nidrā are also almost identical to the components of hypnotherapy. The settling process is crucial to any form of hypnosis, and the movement of awareness around the body is an effective way to induce trance. The pairs of opposites are a classic trance deepener. The difference between yoga nidrā and hypnosis is that in yoga nidrā you guide yourself into the space of trance, even if you are following instructions. It is your own inner voice that carries you through the practice, so you only ever engage with what is perfect for you right now.

▶ *Need to know*

Am I in a trance when I practice yoga nidrā?

Yes. Trance is a perfectly natural phenomenon, and we enter and leave different forms of trance many times during any 24-hour period. In yoga nidrā, we cultivate conscious awareness of this process.

Curiosity is a powerful way to approach the seventh ingredient. Savoring the flavor of what you placed at the start of the practice can be as easy as just asking questions. The wisdom that arises at the end of the practice of yoga nidrā may be cognitive, as it was for Adam, or completely embodied, as it was for Mel. The easiest way to explore either option is to remain curious and to welcome the benefits of rest that may arise at the end of the practice. The following series of inquiries guide you into this openly curious space so that you can welcome the gift of whatever form of wisdom may arise.

Special ingredient: Keeping curious

Returning to welcome the space of simply being

Flip back to the third serving suggestion in Chapter 3 ('Ways to inner listening #3 – Embodied intuition,' on page 79). Feel into your favorite settling ingredient, and softly allow your breath to travel down from head to toe, then ask yourself these questions as you read. Then, feel free to listen to audio track 7.0 (see listing page 2).

◆ If an intention arose for this practice at the start, I wonder, how would it be to return to that intention now?

◆ How about if I were to give myself permission to receive the intuitive wisdom that arises in the deepest nourishment of rest? Where in the spaces inside the body would this wisdom be resting right now?

Then cycle again through each question in 'Ways to inner listening #3.'

As you ask the questions, rest your hands on each part of the body in turn, inquiring into your feeling sense with kindly curiosity.

Follow the inquiries with this encouragement to yourself:

> Whichever aroma or taste,
> whatever sight, touch, or sound,
> whatever place, or person,
> whichever creature or plant,
> whoever or whatever it is
> that brings me even the tiniest piece of joyful delight to recall –
> I invite the memory of that experience to be present
> with gladness within me now.
> I soak up whatever joy that recollection evokes,
> and I let that joy nourish me now in every cell.

Externalize and finish the practice with your favorite flavors. Palming (page 71) would be an excellent exit strategy here, as would the 21-point exit process for sensory reconnection (page 143).

Chapter 8

Externalizing Awareness

Preparing to complete your natural process of yoga nidrā

*as tidal currents circle now
our rhythms of deep rest
move toward cyclic completion
of another nidrā phase –
we are conscious of the land now
waking shallows where we drift –
quiet waves caress the shoreline of the hypnopompic state
floating yoga nidrā dreamers on to this awakening shore
where the liminal encounter of the place where sea meets land
is our space to feel the nidrā waves retreating to the deep*

O f all the ingredients in the nidrā recipes, this is one of the most important to get right.

When we reach the end stages of the practice, we may not be able to leave immediately. Because yoga nidrā is a cyclical process, it can sometimes take a few attempts to find our way out. It's like moving through a revolving door. We may be in the lobby of externalizing awareness, ready to depart from the building of the practice. Although we may enter the revolving door that leads to the outside world, intending to make a rapid exit, we can instead find ourselves slowly spinning around inside this revolving door for several revolutions before we can find our way out. If this happens, we may need to cycle past the main exit several times or return to the lobby and wait for the next circuit of the revolving door before we get outside the building. What to do when we finally leave the building is covered in the next chapter.

▶ *Need to know*

I can't remember anything I heard. How do I know if I am doing this right?

There isn't any way to do yoga nidrā 'wrong.' Each practice is your own experience, and however it turns out is perfect. There is no need to worry about whether you are doing it right. You are just being in the state of awareness which is yoga nidrā, and that is more than enough.

Why is this ingredient included at this point in the process?

Simply put, if we don't include the externalizing of awareness at this stage, then we will not be ready to leave the space of yoga nidrā. It can feel very disturbing to bump up against the end of the practice without sufficient notice that closure is coming. The process of externalizing may need to take the same length of time – or longer – than it took for us to enter the practice in the first place.

Tasting the combinations of flavors of all nine ingredients in the recipe of yoga nidrā can be like having a very long and delicious meal, with lots of different courses. Even when you think you have eaten the final mouthful, there may still be sweet treats to taste. You may go for seconds, or even thirds, or perhaps that final slice of pie is too delicious to resist. Even after dessert is over, there may still be coffee and liqueurs – or even a wafer-thin mint.

Yoga nidrā makes you hungry

All these food metaphors are quite deliberate, and not just because this is a yoga nidrā cookbook. To their surprise, many people discover that they feel ravenously hungry at the end of yoga nidrā. It genuinely takes a lot of energy to rest and daydream. It can be very useful to have a small snack to help you externalize your awareness. We recommend dates, figs, chocolate, or your favorite sweet treat to awaken you through your taste buds!

Here are two tried and tested recipes for effective externalizing.

Externalizing recipe #1

Tune in to the rhythmic breath exit process

This is an excerpt from the tail end of the rhythmic nidrā song in the introduction, specially divided into nine distinct parts, so you can check the gradual process of re-externalizing awareness to the outside world.

Flip back to the rhythmic nidrā song (page 26) and have it ready to read from ingredient 8 to the end. First, read the following instructions to yourself, pausing after each one. If you prefer, you can listen to audio track 8.0 (see listing on page 2).

Connect to the suggested responses, feeling the process of returning to everyday alertness:

1. Resting here the breath is signal to the way to be
    [feel and hear a louder breath]

2. four seasons of this breath are cycling now in perfect time:
    [notice the four parts of the breath in, pause, out, pause]

3. breath in, breath out, breaths in between,
    [ease your breath through the nose, noticing still points between the movements of inhale and exhale]

4. now every breath that moves
    [gently increase the volume of the breath]

5. is felt in all the places where this body meets the earth.
    [consciously notice the places between body and floor beneath]

6. All surfaces beneath me and the sounds of breathing here
    [let out a sigh]

7. are the bridges I can cross now to return to 'every day.'

 [sigh again and maybe yawn]

Then continue with the rest of the rhythmic nidrā practice, following through from externalizing to finish.

Notice how you feel at the end of this externalizing process.

Next time you listen to the rhythmic nidrā song, set your timer for five minutes longer than the recording, and take the time to repeat this externalizing practice twice. Notice if you are more alert than usual afterward.

▶ Need to know

Lots of random thoughts come to me in yoga nidrā. How do I stop them?

Let them come! This is a common experience in yoga nidrā. There is no need to control the thoughts in yoga nidrā because watching them arise is part of the practice.

Externalizing recipe #2

Give yourself more time! A 21-point exit process for sensory reconnection

This recipe deliberately gives you many options to return to the resting state. First read through the process, just as you sit here, becoming aware of your shifting attention.

Cue up the long yoga nidrā audio track and set a timer to finish 10 minutes after the end of the recording.

In the buffer time between the end of the recording and the timer going off, notice your answers to the many inquiries about your readiness to complete the rest cycle. Alternatively you may listen to audio track 8.0 (see listing page 2) that includes these inquiries.

And now, as we come toward the end of this process, it's time to prepare to get ready to leave this state of awareness that is yoga nidrā.

First, conduct some simple inquiries:

1. What can I hear now in the spaces outside this resting body?

2. Is the sound of this breath audible, even if it is very, very quiet?

3. Does the exhale sound different from the inhale?

4. How would it be now to invite the sound of this breath to become a little louder, a little more audible?

5. How about letting the sound of that increasingly louder breath be my bridge to cross back to a more everyday state of awareness?

6. And now, can I notice the movements that accompany this slightly larger breath, the movements of my chest and belly?

7. And along with these movements that accompany my breath, can I notice now the meeting points between my body and the surface beneath?

8. Which parts of my resting body are now touching the surface beneath?

9. And feeling these movements of my breath, and the meeting points between the body and the surface beneath, can I sense the places where the clothes and the covers touch my skin, as well as the surface beneath?

Next, take a moment to reconnect with sensory input:

10. What different temperatures and textures can I feel now on my skin?

11. How does the touch of the air feel upon my eyelids?

12. What can I see through my closed or resting eyelids?

13. And how about my lips? Can I feel the meeting place between my upper and lower lips?

14. And what can I taste now inside my mouth?

15. Encouraging reminder: 'I know that I am resting here in this place now, feeling all these things.'

16. And now I have a choice to make. I ask myself: Am I feeling like I really don't want to move? Am I really done with this? Am I ready to come out?

17. I ask myself: Do I need more time? Do I feel I need to rest a little longer?

18. If I feel I need to rest a little longer, I shall do that. I ask again: Am I rested enough to complete this practice?

Be sure to give yourself heartfelt permission to cycle back into even a few more moments of resting.

19. If I still feel the need for further rest, then I can repeat the practice again or just rest here in this place until I feel ready to arise.

20. If I feel the need to rest longer but am no longer comfortable in the original position, I can roll to the side and rest in the recovery position, or whatever posture feels comfortable for another few minutes or until I feel ready to move.

21. Encouraging reminder: There is no need to rush, I can take my time.

Kindness and patience are the crucial ingredients to ensuring that you are completely externalized, ready to complete the cycle of practice.

Having taken our time to externalize attention, we are now ready to head into Chapter 9 to finish the cycle of your yoga nidrā process.

Chapter 9

Finishing the Practice

Completions, closures, and comparisons

awakening from nidrā –
tides of sleep pull far away
as we rest upon the waking shore of this arriving day –
after rising from our resting
may we be strong and kind –
to be useful and of service here to all who need us now

How do you feel at the end of a yoga nidrā practice? You cannot really savor the flavor of the recipe until after the process is complete. The nature of the exit process determines which flavors remain with us, what benefits we take away. Yoga nidrā can be such a potent experience that it is important to be able to exit from the practice completely and thoroughly. Every method of yoga nidrā always concludes with clear completion instructions marking the end of the practice to ensure that we don't go driving down the road in a state of deeply relaxed communion with the cosmos.

▶ *Need to know*

How long does it take to come around after yoga nidrā practice?

It's varies. Usually after a 15- or 20-minute practice, most people tend to return to alertness within just a few moments, whereas it takes longer to return to the everyday state after lengthier practices. Anything over half an hour can leave you feeling a bit groggy for up to 10 minutes, and after a practice of 40 minutes or more, you may feel a bit spacey for up to a quarter of an hour. But if you are quite tired, even a very short practice can invite you into a sleepy state from which it can feel difficult to awaken. If you are really buzzing before you begin your practice, you can pop straight back into full alertness even after a 45-minute yoga nidrā. With practice, most people tend to become swifter at transitioning both into and out of yoga nidrā experiences, however long they are.

This chapter focuses on exit and completion strategies to finish the practice efficiently so that you can take the synergistic benefits of all the ingredients along with you. In Chapter 2, we included some key basic practices for ensuring that you can leave the practice of yoga nidrā safely and effectively. In this chapter, we add further closure elements.

Serving suggestion: Completion

Choose your favorite yoga nidrā recording, or listen to audio track 9.0 (see listing on page 2).

Set your timer to go off five minutes after the end of the recording.

Before you start listening, flip back to the nine basic ingredients for yoga nidrā exits in Chapter 2 (page 70) to remind yourself of the simple natural movements to awaken.

When you get to the end of the recording, and before the timer goes off, feel your way through whatever ingredients you can easily recall from Chapter 2, then try working through the following sequence of inquiries and encouragements to find what works best for you. Once you've encountered them in this sequence, we invite you to be playful and welcome whichever you find most effective.

1. I can count up, from one to nine, and when I get up to nine, I'll be completely awake and alert.

2. I can count up from one to nine, one breath for each number – one – two – three – four – five – six – seven – eight – and nine.

3. To complete this practice, I affirm to myself: I have been resting in the experience of yoga nidrā; I have been resting in the experience of yoga nidrā; I have been resting in the experience of yoga nidrā.

4. Open and close the eyes.

5. Screw the eyes up tight, then open the eyes wide.

6. Blink rapidly.

7. Rub the palms of the hands together and 'palm' the eyes, resting warm hands over closed eyes, slowly opening eyes to look into the darkness

created by the palms of the hands, and then gently removing the hands from the eyes.

8.   Rub soles of feet together.

9.   Self-massage face, hands, and feet.

When you are good and ready to finish the practice, remind yourself:

> *This practice of yoga nidrā is now complete;*
> *this practice of yoga nidrā is now complete;*
> *this practice of yoga nidrā is now complete.*

Some nidristas enjoy completing the closure with gladness. Try these closing thankful reminders, and see how they feel to you:

> *I thank myself for choosing to resource myself.*

> *I give thanks that I have been able to restore my rhythmic cycles by taking the time to rest in yoga nidrā.*

> *I am grateful for the immense privilege that I have today: the freedom to choose what I want to do with my time.*

Nidrista story: Rising up rested!

To rest in yoga nidrā can be seen as an act of resistance to the patriarchy and its capitalist 'grind culture' that prizes being overworked as a virtue. 'Rise up rested!' is the powerful call from US feminist yoga nidrā trainer Karen Brody, author of Daring to Rest. *Karen encourages women to reclaim the power of their rested selves. Learn more about the Daring to Rest Academy in the resources section at the end of the book.*

Especially after a longer practice, you may find the following options helpful.

Special recipe: 13 wriggles to awaken

These work best in time with your breath and are all easy to do lying down. Do as many or as few as you have time for.

1. Tuck chin down to chest, lift chin, and yawn.

2. Turn head to one side and then the other, yawning on the turns.

3. Drop right ear down to right shoulder and bring head back to center; repeat on left side.

4. Squeeze both shoulders tightly up to ears and then drop shoulders down away from ears.

5. Straighten and bend both arms.

6. Reach both arms up above head, interlock fingers, stretch from side to side.

7. Cross arms around chest and hug tight, then stretch out arms; change cross and repeat.

8. Squeeze and release bum muscles.

9. Bend both knees, press soles of feet into surface beneath, and alternately arch and flatten lower back.

10. Hug knees into belly, stretch out legs, pushing into heels.

11. Hug knees into belly, rest palms of hands gently on knees, and rock from side to side.

12. Keeping hands on knees, with knees apart, circle the knees around to massage lower back.

13. Alternately curl and stretch the toes.

▶ Need to know

I fall asleep during yoga nidrā and never hear anything, but I always come back when I hear the instruction to complete the practice. Have I actually been doing yoga nidrā or have I been asleep?

You have been practicing yoga nidrā because if you had been asleep you would not have heard the instruction to complete the practice, and you would still be asleep. You need to be resting at a certain level of awareness to notice the instruction to return from the practice. You may not be cognitively aware of hearing the instructions, but at another level, your consciousness is responding to the guidance, because you are practicing yoga nidrā and not sleeping.

Serving suggestions for being fully refreshed and alert after yoga nidrā

1. Before you begin, prepare a favorite beverage (warm or cool) and place it in a sealed cup, flask, or bottle by your side ready for you to sip when you awaken.

2. Place a favorite treat within reach for when you complete the practice. Dates, figs, chocolate, or fruits are good, but whatever makes you salivate in anticipation of each taste is perfect.

3. Have within reach your favorite smell to inhale as you awaken. It can be as simple as just a sprig of lavender or an orange to sniff, or perhaps an uplifting aromatherapy oil such as rosemary or citrus oil, or a few drops of your favorite cologne, or agua de Florida if you prefer.

> *to savor doing nothing is the essence of this dish*
> *an antidote to striving –*
> *an act of humble power*
> *to reclaim your right to conscious rest –*
> *reclaim your right to be*
> *in right rhythm with the world that turns*
> *beneath your resting heart*

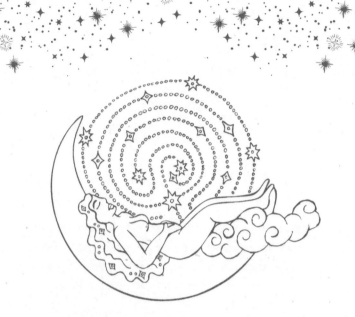

Part II

MAKING YOGA NIDRĀ YOUR OWN

*Now that you have tasted all nine ingredients, you
can appreciate how their unique combination
in a sequenced cyclical process is what
makes the yoga nidrā recipe so unique.*

*Now you are ready to start making
the practice truly your own.*

Chapter 10

Techniques to Practice Natural Yoga Nidrā Solo

You've now tasted all the delicious individual flavors of yoga nidrā and savored how they combine into recipes for restfulness. Even more restful is to simply embody this process, through solo practice, without the need for any instruction from outside. This chapter guides you through the process of cooking 'off book' without the need to check in with the recipe. With repetition, you grow in confidence to measure out your own ingredients and cook up your own special recipes. Solo nidrā truly frees you to make the practice your own, to embody naturally your own uniquely restful way to be.

Natural yoga nidrā memory games

Now that you have savored the complete natural cycle of yoga nidrā, it's time for some natural yoga nidrā memory games. Here are two easy ways to remember the nine ingredients of yoga nidrā more in your body than in your mind. All you need for these little games is a finger and the following diagram.

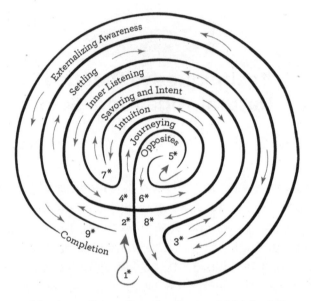

Nine ingredients of a natural yoga nidrā labyrinth

Recipe for the first cycle

Three-breath, easy finger trace around the natural yoga nidrā labyrinth

It's helpful to do this three times, keeping your fingertip on the paper for the entire journey. Briefly pause each time you change direction.

1. Start with your fingertip at the preparation point marked #1 and inhale.

2. As you breathe out, swiftly and lightly trace the whole journey of the labyrinth all the way to the center. Keep your fingertip on the paper for the entire journey, pausing each time you change direction.

3. When you get to the center, inhale, and then as you exhale, trace your finger back out, moving around all the circuits until you get out.

Notice the rhythmic process that circles you into the center of this image and then guides you back to the place where you began, just like the cyclical process of yoga nidrā. Maybe notice the names of all the ingredients on the way in and on the way out of the labyrinth.

Recipe for the second cycle

Nine-breath, easy finger trace around the natural yoga nidrā labyrinth

1. Place the tip of your finger at star point 1 and exhale into this the moment of preparing to begin your process of yoga nidrā – you are claiming this moment for the radical act of rest.

2. Trace your fingertip up the star point 2 and inhale. This is the place where you begin settling into your process of yoga nidrā – resourcing the body of rest. Slowly, as you exhale, trace this circuit of the labyrinth up and around to the right, coming to rest at star point 3.

3. Inhale here at star point 3. Pause in this moment of inner listening and/or inviting intuitive intention – choosing your flavor of yoga nidrā for now. As you breathe out, trace the fingertip all the way up and back over to the left until you come to rest at star point 4.

4. Pause to inhale at star point 4. This is the moment to begin welcoming attention around the body – journeying through places and spaces. As

you exhale, trace the fingertip around the next smaller circuit to the right until you come to rest at star point 5.

5. Pause to inhale at star point 5 in the heart of the yoga nidrā labyrinth. This is the moment for playing with paradox and integration – inviting pairs of opposites. Exhale as your fingertip changes direction, tracing left over the small loop to carry your fingertip down to star point 6.

6. Pause to inhale at star point 6, connecting to imaginative capacity – feeling into sensory and extrasensory knowing. As you exhale, trace the circuit to the left that brings you to star point 7.

7. Pause at star point 7 with an inhale, returning your attention to the taste of inner listening and/or inviting intuitive intention – savoring your flavor of yoga nidrā now. Then exhale as your fingertip traces all the way back around to the right to rest at star point 8.

8. Take another inhale as you pause at star point 8, externalizing awareness – preparing to complete your process of yoga nidrā. As you exhale, circle your fingertip up and over to the left in the outer circuit of the labyrinth until you arrive at star point 9.

9. Inhale one last time, completing the natural cycle of your process – returning to everyday attention with a final exhale.

Notice the names of all the ingredients on the way in and on the way out of the labyrinth. Maybe, if you do this again, become aware of the very simple relationship between the directions of the circuits and the ingredients; perhaps notice how the settling process and the invitation for intent both guide you toward the center, whereas the savoring of intent and the externalizing process both carry you back out.

Tracing the nine ingredients of yoga nidrā through this simple little labyrinth is a simple way to understand the natural, cyclical process of yoga nidrā. If you have already learned another form of yoga nidrā with a different number of elements, and you wish to use this labyrinth model for practicing or sharing, feel free to add in the elements with which you are already familiar. There is space along the circuits to include additional ingredients or to mix in your own special flavors and tastes.

Nine days to your yoga nidrā practice in a voice you can trust: Your own

This progressive series of nine exercises is designed to help you effortlessly recall all nine ingredients in the natural cycle of yoga nidrā so you can eventually practice on your own without the need for a recording. The process combines cognitive learning (studying the ingredients in the relevant chapter) and embodied knowing (listening to and guiding the practice for yourself).

Embodied knowing: Effortlessly recalling your yoga nidrā recipes

This process is based upon how we train yoga nidrā teachers. In our courses, the most important foundation is embodied knowledge of the yoga nidrā process. It is not possible to guide others in this practice with any authenticity unless you can guide yourself easily, without listening to an external voice. In each consecutive day of the training session, just like in the first nine chapters of this book, we focus on a different element, giving people the chance to taste it and feel how it relates to the rest of the recipe. Although the whole facilitator training may last for weeks or months, it initially takes only nine or 10 sessions for people to develop basic confidence with the nine ingredients in our simple recipe for the process of yoga nidrā.

This is a nine-step program that can take as long as you like. It might take you more than nine days to get to the place where you can easily guide yourself in the practice of yoga nidrā without any sense of effort, but, however long it takes, you can proceed gradually through the following simple process, adding an extra flavor each time. If you find you are losing your way, just return to the previous day's step (and the previous chapter) and focus on what you already know. In this way, you build an authentic sense of trust with yourself and with your experience of the cycles of this practice.

▶ *Need to know*

Do I need to actively listen to every instruction and do exactly what I am told?

No. Simply keep a soft and easy connection to the voice. The experience of listening in yoga nidrā is not intended to be active or effortful, but rather relaxed and effortless. There is no need to feel obliged to comply with all the suggestions being made by the facilitator. They are invitations you may follow if you feel that they support your experience of effortless being. If there are any instructions that don't land well with you, simply don't follow them. Let them pass you by and don't engage with them.

Don't be in a rush; this is a skill for life. Grow your embodied knowledge of each ingredient one at a time. Gradually only add the next one as you feel confident. Be excessively gentle with yourself. Repeat each step as often as you need. Meanwhile, continue to listen to the full practice on recordings as often as you like, knowing that each repetition is deepening your own embodied knowledge of the practice.

Making the practice your own: Embodied knowing

An easy way to build embodied knowledge is to sandwich the prerecorded practice with your own self-guided version of the ingredients and gradually empty out the middle 'prerecorded' place until you don't need it all. It's a bit like working with a written recipe, always checking the amounts and the method, until you have done it so often you can cook without the recipe in front of you because you know it so well. This process works best if you listen to the same recording each time. We recommend 'A rhythmic yoga nidrā to remind me how to rest' as a simple short option, or the sequence of audio tracks 10.1–10.8 specially created to support you in making the practice your own (see listing on page 2).

The following pages shows a nine-stage plan to gradually replace the prerecorded practice with your own self-guided practice.

Please remember, there is no rush. Take as long as you like. The stages in this plan do not have to be followed on consecutive days.

Stage 1: Owning the start and the end

Prepare and settle into the process. Assemble your resources (time, space, props). Give yourself five or 10 minutes to get comfortable. Turn on the recording of your choice. Audio tracks 10.1 through 10.8 are a series of simplified, stage by stage audios specially designed to support you in this process (see listing on page 2), or you can pick your own favorite recording with which to work. Listen in. When it's over, repeat the finishing process for yourself, adding in palming (Chapter 2) to ensure you are fully alert.

Stage 2: Settling yourself

Repeat stage 1 but add in a deeper settling, with breath and physical adjustment (Chapter 2). Do this *before* you turn on the recording of your choice. When it's over, repeat the externalizing process for yourself, adding in some additional finishing practices to ensure you are fully alert (Chapter 9).

Stage 3: Inviting the inner guide to speak

Continue to use the self-guided ingredients you included in the previous two stages, but this time, take a minute or two to do some inner listening once you are settled. Invite an intention for your own practice to arise (Chapter 3), asking yourself: As I recall this recipe, could I give myself permission to listen to the inner guiding voice? Do this *before* you turn on the recording. As you listen to the voice, effortlessly invite your own inner guiding voice to be a silent echo of the invitations that you hear from the external voice. Don't be fierce about it. Just let your own inner voice echo fragments of what you hear, every so often, wherever there is space. When the recording is over, repeat the externalizing process for yourself (Chapter 8), adding in some additional finishing practices to ensure you are fully alert (Chapter 9).

Stage 4: Finding your own way around

The main new ingredient now is to welcome attention around the body, starting at the head and ending at the feet. Review what you learned in Chapter 4, then choose a recording that has the same rotation as the one you have studied in this. Go through the same process as stage 3, and then, before you start listening to the recording, simply breathe your attention all the way down your body, exhaling from crown of head to toes and inhaling back up again at whatever pace seems comfortable. Do this nine times before you turn on the recording. During the recording, let the internal voice naturally and effortlessly echo the external voice every so often, especially during the movement of awareness around the body. Be gentle about it. When the recording finishes, repeat the same movement of breath up and down the body as part of your externalizing process for yourself, adding in some additional finishing practices to ensure you are fully alert (Chapter 9).

Stage 5: Knowing and not knowing at the same time

Integrating paradox is the main focus today, specifically the pair of opposites 'knowing and not knowing.' Reread Chapter 5 and use the same recording that you listened to yesterday. Go through the same processes as in stage 4, including breath up and down the body and the inner voice. Before you start listening to the recording, take a moment to be aware of the silent voice within that has been guiding you so far, and all the sounds outside, including the voice you are about to hear. Invite for your own inner voice of guidance to be heard *at the same time* as you listen to the voice on the recording.

When the recording finishes, repeat the movement of attention around the body as part of your externalizing process for yourself just as you did yesterday, but before you complete the practice, simply take time to review which flavors feel familiar and which ones still taste strange. Can you welcome the strange and the familiar at the same time? Only if you feel the need, add some additional finishing practices to ensure you are fully alert (Chapter 9).

Stage 6: Ignoring part of the recording

By now, the process of self-guiding the first five stages is probably becoming familiar, so you can begin to use intuitive visualization to help you embody your knowing. (First, review what you learned about this ingredient in Chapter 6). Then go through all the same self-guiding processes as in stage 5. Turn on the recording, and when you get to the sixth step, the space of inviting intuition (or visualization), simply tune out whatever is being said. Just ignore it. Replace it with your own vivid sense of how it feels to be practicing yoga nidrā in your own inner voice, maybe seeing yourself doing this or feeling it happening, as if you have already remembered how to do it. When the recording finishes, do the same as you did on stage 5, but just as you get to the finish place, reflect: Yes, I have been doing this; I can feel that I have been in this process of yoga nidrā.

Stage 7: Intuitive intention empowers you

Today you can harness the natural cycle of the yoga nidrā process to assist you in guiding the practice for yourself. Repeat the guidance for stage 6. On your way out of the process, when you come to the invitation for intuitive intention (ingredient 7), simply savor your own flavor of yoga nidrā now by repeating: I have been listening to the inner guiding voice. I have been practicing yoga nidrā. I have been guiding myself all the way through. I know all the ingredients, and I know the recipe now.

Stage 8: Becoming free of the external guide

As you prepare to complete your process of embodying recall of yoga nidrā, repeat today all the self-guided preparation and settling processes, going through the same procedure as on stage 7. This is the last day of using the recording, and the instruction today is very simple. When you turn on the recording, just ignore it.

Simply use the recording as a series of cues to hear your own inner guiding voice encouraging you through the practice. You will of course be able to hear the voice of the recording, but now you can relate to it as a helpful guide at your side, reminding you what you already know. When you hear the invitations, respond to them as if they were coming from your own inner guidance.

Flip the script of stage 3, where you let your own inner voice be a silent echo of the voice you could hear on the recording. Now simply hear the recorded voice as if it were an external echo of your inner voice, reminding you that you already know this. This can be quite hypnotic, so once the recording stops, be very sure to give yourself plenty of time to repeat the externalization process and add in your favorite wake-up techniques (Chapter 9).

Stage 9: Stepping into freedom

This stage completes the cycle of your process, so today, simply don't turn on the recording when you start the practice. Keep it ready in case you change your mind (which is fine), but just be curious to see what happens. Replace the recording with a timer and make a choice.

Either set the timer for 27 minutes (or however long your chosen recording is), and settle down to cycle through the whole yoga nidrā process, guided by your inner voice until the timer goes off at the end.

Or set the timer for three minutes. If you go for the three-minute option, each time the timer goes off, press 'Repeat' and move on to the next stage. If you haven't finished the previous one, no worries, just carry on with what you are doing to your satisfaction and start the timer again when you are ready. Some ingredients take longer to cook than others, so this is just a rough guide.

Cycle through all eight stages, or as many of them as you can effortlessly recall, and either see if you can get all the way to the end of the 27-minute timer or see how many three-minute runs you need to get to the end of the recipe.

If you don't like the feeling of either of these experiences, you can always turn the recording back on. If you have chosen the three-minute timer option, then you can also simply ignore the timers and let the process run in its own sweet time. This multiple timer process is unlikely to bring you into the deep states of relaxation that you would get if you just lay back and listened to your recording, but it has the immense benefit of enabling you to track the nine different ingredients as they naturally arise from your previous experiences. You will at least learn what you can recall and see what you have forgotten. It's all good.

You can play the game another way later. This is not the most subtle way to use your timer – it's just the stepping-stone between listening to the recording, listening to your own inner guide, and moving into a wordless experience of yoga nidrā.

To get friendlier with your timer, see the special recipes on page 170. You may also wish to taste a wordless practice (see audio track 12.0 listing on page 2).

You will notice that no matter what flavors are being added to the mix, each step always includes ingredients 1 and 2 (preparation and settling) as well as 8 and 9 (externalization and finish). These are the key ingredients, which is why they are repeated in every session so that you can gain an embodied knowledge of what processes work to settle you and what you need to do to externalize your awareness. This is the bread that makes the sandwich. There is no sandwich without the bread.

You may find it helpful to record progressively more 'empty' yoga nidrā recordings, with quiet gaps that give you space and time to integrate your own embodied knowledge of the ingredients as you get familiar with them. We've gathered a series of 'empty vessel' recordings for this purpose on our website if you feel they would be helpful to hear. You'll find the link to these audio tracks in the resources section at the end of the book. Once you've worked through this series of the nine-ingredient recollection processes, you are ready to move on to the next special recipes that do not use any recordings, just your trusty timer.

Making friends with your external timer to cultivate trust in your own inner timer

Many people worry that if they begin to self-guide their own processes of yoga nidrā, they will simply not wake up at the end. A timer can support you in cultivating trust with your own inner timer so that you will always awaken at the end of the process your internal guide is facilitating. Persistent playfulness with self-guiding nidrās and knowing that you have the back-up of the outside timer will help you learn to trust the cyclical wisdom in your body that always knows just when you need to wake up – because in the end, with practice you will always find yourself awakening just before the timer goes off.

The ninth day of the detailed recipe in embodied knowing introduced the idea of using a timer to replace a recording.

Here are three more helpful ideas to use timers to assist your self-guided practice of yoga nidrā.

1. If you are using a recording, before you begin listening to it, set a timer to end five minutes after the recording finishes. This helps you relax into knowing that if you do not immediately come around at the end of the recording, the timer will awaken you five minutes later. It also gives you the opportunity to self-guide your own externalization and finish practices.

2. If you are aiming to self-guide a 15-minute practice, set a timer for eight minutes at the start of the process. The timer will go off around the time you reach ingredient 5 in the recipe and will helpfully remind you that you are over halfway through. All you need do is press 'Repeat' and then continue to the end of the practice, with a minute to spare.

3. If you want to do an early morning yoga nidrā, use your snooze button as a timer. Before you go to sleep, set the snooze interval for 20 minutes. Then set the alarm for 21 minutes before you need to wake up. In the morning, after the alarm goes off, either start the yoga nidrā recording – or even better, self-guide a yoga nidrā process – knowing that the snooze alarm will awaken you at the end, and you can go into your day relaxed and refreshed.

Now that you have begun to make yoga nidrā your own, we are ready to start cooking up special occasion recipes for specific purposes.

Each of the next three chapters is devoted to three specific applications of yoga nidrā, starting with yoga nidrā to help you go to sleep.

Chapter 11

Yoga Nidrā to Improve Sleep

resting on the nidrā sea
sleep draws us down within
to sink beneath the surface
of this waking consciousness
until we rest upon the waking shore of this arriving day

We all need our sleep. For most people, this is between seven to nine hours each night. If we regularly sleep fewer than seven hours a night, we are sleep deprived, and every aspect of physical health deteriorates rapidly.[20] Lack of sleep shortens our life. Tiredness makes us more prone to obesity, heart disease, and diabetes.[21] Most people are not getting enough sleep,[22] and inadequate, or poor-quality sleep severely damages mental balance and makes us more prone to anxiety and depression.[23]

Thankfully, yoga nidrā is well known to support both initial sleep onset and returning to sleep if we awaken in the night.[24] This chapter shares three simple effective yoga nidrā techniques to manage insomnia and encourage healthy sleep cycles. You'll also learn how the daytime settling processes you experience in your yoga nidrā nest can be cultivated to enable you to drift off to sleep easily (and drift *back* into sleep easily) if you wake up in the middle of the night. Because yoga nidrā is a meditation upon the process of falling asleep, many people confuse the 'yogic sleep' of yoga nidrā with ordinary sleep. Before we dive into the practicalities of how yoga nidrā can improve sleep, it's important to understand how sleep works and why yoga nidrā is not a sleep replacement.

▶ *Need to know*

I experience depression/anxiety. Is it safe to practice yoga nidrā?

Very possibly yes. It all depends on the nature, cause, and duration of your experiences of depression or anxiety, and the type of yoga nidrā you practice. Some yoga nidrā practices can alleviate anxiety or depression, but some can aggravate these states. It is important to observe with kindness your own responses. Shorter practices that focus attention on welcoming external sensory input, such as sounds and sensations, are generally more appropriate for depression, whereas longer, more leisurely yoga nidrās with what is known as 'coherent breath,' with equal lengths of inhalation and exhalation, and experiences of balance and grounding are more suitable for anxious people. (See page 202 for a simple recipe to support equivalent breath). The physical resting position is a significant element to adapt the practice to suit you. Additional propping to support the body in side-lying or curling into a fetal position can help manage anxiety, whereas a supported semi-reclining posture with an open chest is likely to be more suitable for depression.

Nidrista Story: Decades of insomnia

For thirty years, Nirlipta was a total insomniac. Unable to get to sleep, he'd lie awake for hours, and then if he did finally drop off, he'd wake up in the middle of the night completely wired, and stay that way until silly o'clock, when he'd drag himself out of bed to face another day exhausted. It all changed when he met yoga nidrā. 'Nidrā transformed my relationship with sleep. First, I made friends with my insomnia, because I felt good about having something to do when I was lying awake in bed. Then I realized what I was practicing in yoga nidrā calmed my frazzled nervous system so I could get back to sleep. That's why I created my Sleep Well with Yoga Nidrā course especially for insomniacs: I know what it's like!' To learn more about Nirlipta's work with insomnia, see the resources section at the end of the book.

Sleep moves in cycles: So does yoga nidrā

The reason yoga nidrā feels so restful is because it mimics the process of cycling through different brain-wave states and sleep stages, just as we do when we are asleep. But it does not give us the amount of rest we need nightly. The science of yoga nidrā's effect on brain waves has been researched since the 1970s.[25] Studies show that, during a 20-minute practice of yoga nidrā, people can cycle through the whole set of brain waves we cycle through at night. The key difference is that, during a full night's sleep, we have multiple sleep cycles, not just one. In addition, these nighttime sleep cycles provide much longer periods of deeply restorative delta waves, both within each sleep cycle and cumulatively throughout the whole night.

▶ *Need to know*

Will practicing yoga nidrā keep me awake at night?

It's more likely to help you sleep better. Practicing yoga nidrā during the daytime or evening can help you feel more relaxed and more consciously aware of your capacity to drop off to sleep. Practicing yoga nidrā is meditating upon the process of falling asleep, and with repetition, we may find that we become better at this process.

Although we experience delta and other brain waves during yoga nidrā, there is simply insufficient time spent in the deeply restful state during one practice for it to *replace* the need for normal sleep. (In the next chapter, you'll learn more about the effects of different brain waves.)

It may seem that practicing yoga nidrā makes us feel *as if* we have slept sufficiently, and that we can thus use it to replace sleeping hours, but this is not how the practice works. Yoga nidrā is more like a sleep supplement than a sleep replacement. To understand how the practice can help improve our ordinary sleep, it is helpful to understand natural human sleep cycles and how they get disrupted.

▶ *Need to know*

I keep falling asleep in yoga nidrā. Am I doing it wrong?

There is no way to do yoga nidrā wrong. The whole intention of the practice is to simply rest and *be*, to witness whatever arises without effort or focus, including the process of falling asleep. The practice is effectively a meditation on the act of falling asleep, so if you do go to sleep during the practice, that is fine –it is part of the practice too. So again, it is not possible to get this wrong. Whatever happens is part of your experience of the practice. Because the process of yoga nidrā meets the needs of the practitioner, you may find that if you practice more often, you become less tired and that, in time, you may sleep less during yoga nidrā.

Sleep cycles, sleep stages, and yoga nidrā

It's only relatively recently that sleep scientists identified two forms of sleep: rapid eye movement (REM) sleep and non-rapid eye movement (NREM) sleep.[26] REM is dreaming sleep, when the brain is most active, using the highest amounts of oxygen and calories, whereas during NREM sleep, the brain is resting. We encounter these two different forms of sleep throughout the night in five stages: NREM 1 through 4, and REM. The sequence of these five stages makes one full sleep cycle that lasts about 90 minutes. We usually experience around five or six sleep cycles throughout the night, as you can see from the following hypnogram.

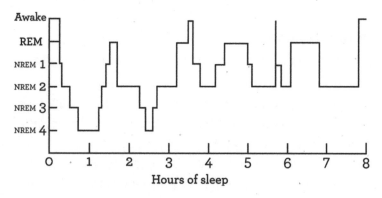

Hypnogram showing the stages of sleep

NREM 1 is light sleep, or hypnagogia. In it, we are sleeping and feel daydreamy, but we also have awareness of our surrounding environment, which is why we sometimes think we are sleeping far less than we are – we can literally be awake and asleep simultaneously. Not too much time asleep is spent here. This is the liminal stage of sleep, and this is the stage we inhabit mostly in yoga nidrā. The most recent research about yoga nidrā to support sleep onset explores how daytime experiences in this stage can help people to settle into deeper sleep at night.[27]

In **NREM 2,** muscles relax more, breathing and heartbeat slows down. Maybe half of the time we are asleep is spent here, with theta wave activity predominant. NREM 2 is when we process most memories from the previous day. We are likely to inhabit this stage of sleep as we settle into yoga nidrā.

In **NREM 3** and **NREM 4,** we experience the deepest rest, least mental activity, and our eyes remain relatively immobile. These two stages typically make up about a quarter of the time spent sleeping, and the most important and longest of these stages occurs in the first phase of our sleep. We may drop into brief periods of these deeply restful states during yoga nidrā.

In healthy sleep cycles, the four stages of NREM are followed by REM sleep, the dreaming phase where the eyes move and the body is partially paralyzed, so that we don't act out our dreams. It is in REM where our brain's energy and oxygen consumption peak, at its most active for the whole 24-hour cycle. A quarter of our time asleep is spent here. We can encounter REM sleep during yoga nidrā, but it is different from experiences we have in nightly sleep.

Just like regular sleep, yogic sleep involves stages of REM and NREM, but in different degrees and duration. In regular REM sleep, our brains are actively engaged in dreaming; but in REM yoga nidrā, our brains are actively engaged in trance. In NREM states in yoga nidrā, we often have the same hallucinatory imagery and sensations, as well as some degrees of physiological rest, just as we get in NREM 1 and 2. It is also possible to experience moments of deeply restorative NREM 3 and 4 during yoga nidrā. A key difference between regular sleep and yogic sleep is that in yoga nidrā, consciousness remains active. Body and mind are deeply resting as if we were asleep, but awareness is present.

Circadian and ultradian rhythms

In addition to the phases of sleep, daily (circadian) and multiple 90-minute ultradian rhythms, rely upon natural light to govern our waking and sleeping cycles. Both the daily ultradian and nightly sleep cycles are approximately 90 minutes long and are usually matched by a shift in the passage of air through the nostrils. Humans also have built-in sleep-regulating mechanisms to aid the balance between sleep and waking hours by signaling our need to sleep through the experience of tiredness.

Adult humans often override these signals with late-night screen time and other forms of digital slavery that keep us awake even when we are exhausted so that we find it increasingly difficult to get to sleep. Regular practice of yoga nidrā can help us to recognize and respond to natural calls for sleep, giving us a reliable way to relax and drift off. In simple terms, yoga nidrā can help us relearn how to respond to natural rhythmic cycles, so we can both awaken full of energy and go to sleep more easily.

Nidrista story: A rested doctor is safer

*In November 2014, following the death of a
sleep-deprived young doctor who crashed her car while
driving home from a night shift, the UK Association of
Anaesthetists and the Royal College of Anaesthetists, in
association with the Faculty of Intensive Care Medicine,
investigated the serious problem of fatigue among their
members. In response to their findings, they produced a
fatigue resource educational pack for doctors. It includes
a very clear instruction: 'Download a yoga nidrā audio
and use it.' They advise that regular practice of yoga
nidrā can support alertness during night shifts and help
avoid fatal car accidents.*[28]

Biphasic sleep

Before we get cooking with the practicalities of how yoga
nidrā can help us get to sleep, it's vital to know that it is
quite natural for humans to sleep in two parts, punctuated
by a period of waking in between. This is called biphasic
sleep, and it is perfectly normal. The expectation that we
should sleep for eight hours uninterruptedly is a very recent
development indeed. Since the invention of electric light
and the Industrial Revolution, natural patterns of human
sleep have been profoundly disrupted by the demands of a
colonial capitalist economic system that requires workers to
remain alert and productive for eight-hour shifts. Insomnia
as a widespread medical issue concept did not exist until
the 1920s. Now, it's officially an epidemic.[29]

Often, what we think of as insomnia is simply a natural remnant of preindustrial human sleep cycles with ancient roots in human evolution. Knowing this can help make sense of our sleeping patterns today as well as make friends both with our evolutionary heritage of naturally arising cycles of sleep and with our own preindustrial patterns of sleeping and waking. Yoga nidrā can be a practical tool to help 21st-century humans improve our sleep under adverse circumstances. Yoga nidrā done in these darkest hours can help us to go back to sleep, but it can also help us with some of our best thinking, insights, and problem-solving (as we explored in Chapter 6).

▶ *Need to know*

I feel more tired after practicing yoga nidrā. Why?

Many people often feel fully refreshed and energized after practicing yoga nidrā, but sometimes the opposite occurs. If you feel more tired at the end of the practice than you did at the start, it is likely that you were unaware of just how deeply exhausted you were before you began. Yoga nidrā can reveal very deep levels of exhaustion and highlight the detrimental effects of years of sleep deprivation. The cyclical process of yoga nidrā can show us just how tired we really are. If this is the case, it can be helpful to do two practices of yoga nidrā back-to-back and drift off to sleep during the first practice as if it were a nap, a chance to catch up on deep rest. Then the second practice can nourish and revive so you are more likely to feel refreshed when you finish.

Another strategy is to practice yoga nidrā first thing in the morning after waking up, when the body is more likely to have a basic level of rest to begin with, so that by the end of the practice you may be sufficiently rested to feel revived.

Philosophical background of yoga nidrā: Multidimensional rest

Understanding the basics of sleep science, circadian rhythms, and the prehistory of biphasic sleep helps us appreciate how and why we sleep (or have trouble sleeping) the way we do. These Western explanations reveal physical and mental issues associated with sleep problems, but there are other important dimensions to our experiences of sleep. The philosophical background of yoga nidrā illuminates these emotional, psychological, and intuitive dimensions of rest and sleep.

One of the big ideas at the heart of yogic philosophy is the understanding that human experience, including the experience of sleep, exists in more than just the material world. Our physical bodies are only one aspect of our reality, and yoga nidrā, like all yoga practices, operates in five dimensions. The other four aspects are: our vitality, our thoughts and emotions, our intuitive and imaginative capacities, and our experience of connection to the source of all.

Clearly, all five of these different capacities are interdependent: It is hard to maintain emotional stability when we are in physical pain, and it is challenging to retain high vitality when we are grieving. The five capacities are not just interconnected; they are also all depleted when we are tired, and physical tiredness is only one part of the problem. The great gift of yoga nidrā is that it can address all these different capacities in a single practice. At the start of every yoga nidrā practice, we not only focus attention upon settling the physical body, but also attend to breath, feelings, thoughts, intuitive capacity, and the awareness that watches all of this.

This multidimensional capacity of yoga nidrā is one of the reasons that it works so well as a support for sleep. When we sleep, it is not just our physical bodies that rest, but also every other aspect of our being. Just as tired bones and muscles recuperate in our sleep, thoughts and emotions take a restful pause as well, while intuitive and creative capacities are nourished. Yoga nidrā systematically induces total relaxation in every dimension of being, not simply the physical, and this is one of the reasons it helps us sleep so well: We are not just physically tired, but emotionally and mentally exhausted too. So the multidimensional practice of yoga nidrā is an effective way to rest deeply in every aspect of being.

Sound good? You don't need to take our word for it. Next time you are tucking up for the night, take time to do these simple exercises and experience it for yourself.

Serving suggestions

Settling deeper into rest

This simple technique is based on the first and second ingredients of yoga nidrā. Try it when you first settle in to go to sleep.

1. Notice all places where the body is touching the surface beneath, and consciously give away the weight down into that surface.

2. Work down from head to feet, noticing contact with the pillow, the bed beneath. It doesn't matter which position you lie in. Adjust if you need to get more comfortable as you work down the body.

3. As you exhale, give the whole weight of each body part into the surface beneath. Feel the surface beneath welcoming the weight of the body. Notice that more of you is in contact with the surface. Repeat as often as you need until the whole weight of the body is held.

Welcoming every part of the body into restful sleep

This uses the fourth ingredient of yoga nidrā to invite sleep to enter the body.

1. After you have settled the body into comfort, consciously and kindly send an invitation to every part of the body to 'welcome rest.'

2. Start at the top of the head and move down – use the itinerary you are most familiar with. Be kind and attentive.

3. The more detail you go into the longer it takes to get down to the toes and the more likely you are to fall asleep. Use the detailed itineraries for journeys of attention around the body in Chapter 4 for ideas.

Settling the body physically, then mentally allowing each part to relax is not just important for establishing comfort. A key benefit of the preparatory and settling ingredients of any yoga nidrā recipe is to make a deliberate separation from the rest of your day. When you settle down into your nidrā nest in the daytime and stop 'doing' as you prepare to rest, you draw very clear boundaries. You learn to draw a line under what went before, then simply rest in yoga nidrā. The more you practice this in the daytime, the easier it will be to do it at night.

Reviewing the day before you sleep

clean the pot of daytime thoughts –
don't sleep with dirty scraps
on the inside of the saucepan
that you cook your dreams within

Consciously reviewing your day and bringing yourself into the present moment is vital in using yoga nidrā to fall asleep and to return to sleep if you wake up in the night. Reviewing the day cleans out the cooking pot of your awareness, removing flavors of the preceding day – it leaves the pot clean for the next ingredients, restful sleep, and dreams.

Special recipe: Cleaning your cooking pot

1. Settle comfortably. Begin by recalling the process of awakening, returning your attention to the moment when you first opened your eyes this morning.

2. Next, simply remember getting up, and see or sense yourself moving through the day, recalling whatever you did.

3. Let this be effortless! Only attend to recollections that come easily. Don't try too hard. Let it be an informal process, inviting memories to pop up in the order they occur. You may focus on individual incidents, or simply invite a general sense of the day's flow.

4. Gradually take yourself right up to the moment when you got into bed, noticing how you feel now after settling. Be aware if you feel any different now than you did when you first got into bed.

5. If you're still wide awake or engaged with ideas from your day, you can repeat the process in reverse, beginning with the present moment and returning awareness back through the day until you come to where you first woke up. If you are still awake, reverse the process again.

Watch the movie of your day without judgment or reflection, simply as a quiet observer. There are two key benefits to this. The first is that it can help you prepare for sleep by filing away the activities of the day, and the second is that doing this practice before you go to sleep tends to give you clearer dreams. Because you have already 'cleaned the pot' of your day's activities before you start cooking up your dreams, you tend to have fewer dreams about daily concerns.

Whether or not you recall your dreams, including a review of the day in your nighttime yoga nidrā practice is a habit well worth cultivating. It enables you more easily to make the transition between daytime activities and nighttime rest.

▶ Need to know

Choose carefully!

Although yoga nidrā can be used successfully to get to sleep or back to sleep, take care to choose a recording designed for sleeping. It is disturbing to use a yoga nidrā recording that brings you close to the onset of sleep, but then hearing a cheery voice at the end telling you to rise up refreshed to carry on with the day. Pick a recording specifically designed *not* to wake you up at the end[30] – or even better, learn to do the practice yourself so you don't need to listen to a recording.

Special recipe: Yoga nidrā in your sleep

A great way to practice self-guiding your yoga nidrā process is to bring it to bed with you.

One of everyone's favorite homework assignments on our teacher trainings is the nightly process of settling yourself to sleep using yoga nidrā. Every night for a week, simply add an extra step from the yoga nidrā before you go to sleep. Because by the time you turn out the light, you've already made time and space to practice, and because you are also likely to have dropped off before you get to the end, that leaves only seven ingredients – one for every day of the week.

Follow the instructions for the ninth stage of the embodied knowing program (page 163) and see if you can stay awake long enough to get to the end. Don't stress about remembering the process verbatim, just welcome whatever you can recall easily. If you are still awake, give it another go. If you wake up in the middle of the night just carry on from where you left off. You won't need to reach for a recording because your inner guide is running the process.

We find that people are more relaxed in this way and less likely to worry about forgetting different ingredients or the order of the recipe. The point is not to develop perfect recall of a script, but to deepen your own embodied knowledge of your response to the ingredients as you cycle through the process.

Nidrista story: Yoga nidrā as a sleep supplement

One-third of UK drivers regularly fall asleep at the wheel in a 'micro-sleep.'[31] It is the most common form of death for lorry drivers. A few years ago, Nirlipta discovered he was experiencing a lot of micro-sleeps on frequent drives to London. He was having difficulty staying awake for the two-and-a-half-hour journey due to an undiagnosed respiratory condition. Realizing this was dangerous, he came up with a plan. He would pull into a service station, recline the seat, and do a seven- or 11-minute yoga nidrā. During the practice, his experience of time was helpfully distorted so that it felt as though he had rested deeply for 45 minutes. Thus refreshed, he would be alert enough to drive safely to his destination and have sufficient energy to teach. Yoga nidrā doesn't replace sleep, but it can supplement the lack of it, and in dire straits, it can keeps things on an even keel – or as Nirlipta found, save your life.

But yoga nidrā is not just all about sleep. There are many other physical and psychological benefits of the practice, including healthier digestion, more comfortable menstruation, and the reduction of pain, anxiety, and stress. In the next chapter, you'll learn how yoga nidrā can effectively manage stress.

Chapter 12

Yoga Nidrā to Relieve Stress and Pain

there is wisdom in forgetting
there is healing in this sleep
there is dropping out of worry when we finally let go
when we let go of our holding on to stay
in wakefulness –
when we rest in yoga nidrā
it invites us to forget –
it invites us to be still now
it invites us to give up
what we think to be important when we're ruled by the belief
that our value is dependent on the work that we can do

'The sleep of the yogis' can be a nourishing supplement to healthy sleep for ordinary humans. But there is more to yoga nidrā than sleep. Sleep and the circadian rhythms and cycles that support it are just one of many cyclical functions vital to human health. Stress itself functions cyclically, and tiredness intensifies our experiences of chronic and acute stress and pain. Our experiences of acute stress and pain are directly related to our responses to everyday stressors in the cycles of our lives.

This chapter shares five simple breathing practices to add to yoga nidrā recipes to relieve stress and pain. You'll learn why and how the restful process of yoga nidrā can build resilience to stressful or painful experiences. Being well rested makes us more resilient because rest supports the healthy rhythmicity of bodily functions.[32] This frees up energy to enable us to respond to stressors from a place of relaxed vitality. The relaxing space of yoga nidrā is an ideal place to use easy breath techniques to restore natural cycles of digestion, menstruation, and relaxation and stress responses.

▶ *Need to know*

Can I practice yoga nidrā after eating?

It depends how much you have eaten and in which position you rest for the practice. Many people drift off to sleep when they practice directly after eating a heavy meal, so it can be preferable to take a short stroll between the end of a large meal and the start of yoga nidrā. After a light meal, yoga nidrā can work very well. Either way, try resting on the left side and keep the practice short, around 15 minutes.

To help us understand how all this works, we first explore the basics of the science behind cyclical patterns of brain-wave activity arising in yoga nidrā. As you read, you'll learn how to use simple breath and body awareness in yoga nidrā to recognize and navigate brain-wave states and other physiological cycles.

Measuring brain waves: Navigating states of being in yoga nidrā

Neuroscientists identify five different states of human brain activity by measuring the electrical impulses generated when brain cells (neurons) communicate. This electrical activity is evident in synchronized oscillations, or vibrations known as brain waves. The five brain-wave states are named after letters in the Greek alphabet: beta, alpha, theta, delta, and gamma. Each brain-wave state has a range of impulses measured in vibrations called hertz. Vibration frequency indicates which brain-wave state is predominant.

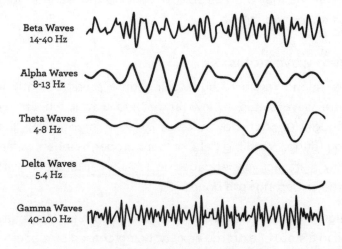

The five brain-wave states

In the following very simplified descriptions of the five brain-wave states, we translate figures into feelings through simple phrases that convey the familiar human experiences of each state. We also highlight when and how these experiences may show up in yoga nidrā. There are simple breath practices for you to try as you read about each state so you can notice the differences between them.

The first step in learning how to manage our different responses to stressors and to de-stressors is to notice what is happening in our body mind. This is the gift of yoga nidrā, which literally gives us time to do nothing but observe ourselves, without judgment, just as we are. If, in the state of yoga nidrā, we can become aware of how certain parts of the process evoke certain brain-wave states, we may then be able to replicate these shifts when we encounter stress.

Beta wave states

We spend much of our waking time predominantly in beta wave states. In low-range beta waves, we can be thoughtful, but not necessarily very productive: 'just cogitating.' Middling beta, or 'beta proper,' is when we are fully alert, actively engaged in tasks or interaction with others: 'Getting stuff done.'

High beta is when we are very focused indeed. We might be in a state of extreme anxiety, being chased by a pack of wolves and running for our lives, or we could be processing new and intense experiences, learning highly complex concepts, or simply being very excited: 'Eeek!' Adrenaline flows and the flight, fight, or freeze reflex is likely to kick in. Our physiology is not intended to function well if we spend too much time continually in high beta states, but the demands of living in an aggressively competitive, industrial, capitalist society put most humans under daily, intolerable stresses that result in almost permanent high beta states.

The problem with living for extended periods in the beta state is that, even though it makes us very tired, many of us become habituated to this level of exhaustion and do not even notice how depleting it is until we stop. Simply lying down, preparing to begin yoga nidrā, just before the practice starts, can give us the pause that we need to notice our beta state.

In the preparatory stage of yoga nidrā, it is possible to notice physical signs indicating we are beginning to relax. As we get horizontal and shift out of hectic, everyday thought patterns, we also may observe changes in breathing and heart rate. It's the feeling of arriving home after a tiring journey, or a long day's work, putting down our bags, taking off our shoes, and feeling an embodied sense of relief. This transitional moment can often be heard as an audible, glad sigh: 'Aaah!'

Simple breathing recipe for transitioning out of beta states during yoga nidrā

As you sit here now, or next time you get ready to practice yoga nidrā, let out a huge sigh – or three. Now yawn. Now yawn again, bigger. And now, close your lips as you sigh. Invite the sigh to become a hum. Continue to hum on each out-breath for as long as you like. There is no need to make a loud or long sound. Just let the humming continue easily as you breathe out. Notice how the whole body responds to the breath and the sound. This simple process can help us transition out of beta state, toward alpha, or at least from high beta into the lower ranges of this brain-wave state. Do not underestimate the immense power of the simple resonance of your own voice inside your body, especially if you are horizontal. When you are ready, let go of this little game, and return to breathing easily as you rest.

Alpha wave states

Alpha waves are slower than beta waves and indicate what is sometimes called a flow state, a place of relaxed effortless ease. It's an experience of being present in the here and now, beyond any sense of deadlines or time pressures. It's a resting place for the mind, in which we experience expanded peripheral awareness of the outside world without having to think too much. We are mentally and physically relaxed, alert but calm: 'I'm here. Just hangin' in the zone.'

As we settle deeper into yoga nidrā, after the first few minutes, alpha waves tend to predominate. Even people who have never done yoga nidrā before are very likely to drop into alpha state soon after the practice starts.[33] This is the substratum of yoga nidrā, and it tends to continue throughout the whole process. As we cycle in and out of other brain-wave states, it is to the alpha state that we return most often. It is here that most people notice a restful state of being simultaneously aware and calmly centered.

> *this is a simple act to make*
> *an easy choice to be*
> *for a space of 20 minutes to be resting quietly –*
> *this body is relieved to stop*
> *the heart can settle now*
> *and the lungs can breathe their fullness*
> *to bring energy to rest*

Nidrista story: Alpha dog chilling

When Swami Rama, founder of the Himalayan Institute, was being wired up to test his brain-wave states as he demonstrated yoga nidrā in a Texas laboratory in 1971, he brought his German shepherd dog along to keep him company during the experiments. He joked that maybe the researchers should connect the dog to the same machines that were testing his master. They did just that and discovered that the dog demonstrated continual alpha waves. It was a very relaxed dog.

Two breathing recipes for sustaining alpha wave states in yoga nidrā

1. As you sit here now, or next time you get ready to practice yoga nidrā, notice sensations of breath arriving and leaving the nostrils. Can you notice the difference between the temperature of the breath coming in and the temperature of the breath going out? Can you feel the movement of breath on the upper lip and inside the nose? That's it. Just notice these sensations. When you are ready, let go of this little game, and just return to breathing easily as you rest.

2. As you sit here now, or next time you get ready to practice yoga nidrā, sigh out a few times through softly parted lips, as if you were breathing onto a mirror to clean it. Feel the sound in the throat as you do this. Then close the lips and feel for the same sensation in the throat. Keep the breath gentle now and keep the same sound that you felt when the lips were open. It may feel as if you have bypassed your nose and are just breathing softly straight into your throat. Keep the throat soft as you maintain this gentle breath at an easy pace. That's it. Just notice these sensations. When you are ready, let go of this little game, and return to breathing easily as you rest. This is the breath that you do every night when you are asleep, and it may feel quite soporific.

Easy breath observation tends to calm both respiratory and heart rates and slow the procession of thoughts, helping you to stay in the alpha zone – in yoga nidrā and in life. This process can help you notice your arrival in the alpha zone and effortlessly sustain your relaxed connection to this state. Often a conscious attentiveness to the breath, a meditative space, quite naturally arises in alpha. Just welcome this pleasant state and observe it. You can also cultivate this experience throughout yoga nidrā, so it is easier to recall the feeling of being in alpha and evoke it again as a positive response to any perceived stressors.

Theta wave states

Theta waves are even slower than alpha waves, creating a threshold place that we often enter during yoga nidrā. Theta also occurs in sleep, mostly in light sleep, when we process new events, file memories, and observe stimuli arising from within rather than from outside.

This is the state in which we daydream; and at night, these are the brain waves in which REM dreaming arises. At both the points in yoga nidrā when we rest in the deepest states of the alpha zone, and at night when we drift into the hypnogogic state, we may notice that we are arriving in the theta wave states.

The characteristic experience of theta state is surreal daydream imagery, feelings, recollections, or thoughts, with an accompanying sense of 'Wow! Cool! It's getting a bit weird in here now.' When we accept that these, often bizarre, images and thoughts are a normal characteristic of this brain-wave state, we can feel at home in the liminality of theta, between consciousness and unconsciousness. Here we can stay, letting intuitive insights arise and observing them, or sinking down deeper within ourselves to rest soundly. Theta state is where creative inspirations, insights, and solutions can arise.

Simple breathing recipe for entering and remaining in theta states

As you sit here now, or next time you get ready to practice yoga nidrā, let your breath travel through the nose. Now watch the inhale and the exhale becoming roughly equal in length. There is no counting involved at all. Just welcome the sense that both inhaling and exhaling feel about the same length. Now, notice the natural pauses at the end of the inhale before exhalation begins, and then the end of the exhalation before the inhale begins. Welcome these pauses naturally without counting or forcing them. This is effortless 'equivalent breathing.' Let it feel balanced and easy as it comes and goes. When you are ready, let go of this little game, and return to breathing easily as you rest.

This technique of equivalent breathing is a useful stress-relief practice for people who have respiratory issues, including chronic obstructive pulmonary disease (COPD), asthma, and breathing issues associated with long Covid. The absence of counting or breath control makes it easily accessible, even if breathing is challenging.

Delta wave states

Delta waves oscillate much more slowly and more powerfully than theta waves. The slower the frequency, the higher the amplitude, so these are the most powerful of all the brain waves. It is here that very deep meditative experiences, NREM 3 sleep, and restorative healing occur. Thoughts slow to a halt. This can be a quiet space beyond dreaming. These brain waves bring us to a wordless space that can't be described while we are in it. When we return from delta wave states, we can sense that we have been 'totally gone.'

In yoga nidrā, this is the place where we can be aware of deeply resting, even noticing, momentarily, that we are not thinking. It is a powerfully peaceful space. All external awareness recedes far into the background as we rest in a spacious state of pure being, not doing. It is very rare to be conscious of this place.

It is here in delta that we can experience the most profound relief from pain and stress. This is the place where deep healing occurs.

▶ *Need to know*

How can I practice yoga nidrā when I am in too much pain to lie still?

One of the challenges of practicing yoga nidrā while in pain is finding a position sufficiently comfortable in which to rest. It is important to acknowledge the presence of pain at the start, and to respect that physical movement during yoga nidrā may be necessary to permit the practice to happen at all. A good strategy is to cycle through two or three different positions, perhaps beginning more upright or seated, then shifting to side-lying, then rolling over toward the end of practice. Kind persistence and respect for changing needs of the body is the best strategy for practicing yoga nidrā in pain. It can be very helpful to precede yoga nidrā by a series of gentle, small movements throughout the body, coordinated with breath awareness to release tension before attempting to find a restful position.

Simple breathing recipe for entering and remaining in delta wave states

As you sit here now, or next time you get ready to practice yoga nidrā, let your breath settle in to an easy pace. Now simply rest your attention in the pause between the end of the next exhale and the beginning of the next inhale. After this, rest your attention in the pause between the next inhale and beginning of the following exhale. You may notice, especially if you try this in yoga nidrā, that the pauses can easily extend into long spaces of just being, without doing. When you are ready, let go of this little game, and return to breathing easily as you rest.

Gamma wave states

Gamma waves are where many different sources of information from different parts of the brain are brought together and processed simultaneously. It is a highly intuitive state of being, connected to higher virtues, such as empathy, altruism, higher cognitive activity, and clear insight. It's the sense of clear recognition: 'Eureka!

I get it!' In gamma wave states, ordinary activities of the mind quieten, and insight arises. Gamma states are often observed in frequent meditators and are the characteristic brain-wave state at moments of creative inspiration or problem-solving.

Simple breathing recipe for inviting gamma wave states

As you sit here now, or next time you get ready to practice yoga nidrā, let your breath settle in to an easy pace. Simply notice the back of your body and the surface upon which it rests. Breathe into it as you exhale. Notice the points of contact between the back body and the surface beneath, then simply rest your attention in the front body and the space around it. Inhale into this space. Notice the air and space around the front body and above the head. Alternate easily between noticing the back body on the exhale and the front body on the inhale. Softly exhale attention into the back, then softly inhale attention into the front. Back, then front. And now, very gently, can you notice both front and back at the same time? Can you rest your attention in the two places at the same time and just notice what you notice? What happens now? When you are ready, let go of this little game, and return to breathing easily as you rest.

Multiple brain-wave states throughout the cyclical process of yoga nidrā

Different brain waves can arise simultaneously during yoga nidrā. An individual encounter with yoga nidrā cannot be defined as predominantly one brain-wave state or another. Neither can a linear process be traced straight from beta through to delta. As we practice, we can be aware of resting at the boundaries between the relaxed state of alpha and the surreal boundaries of theta. We can bring some beta-like observation skills to the experiences of theta. There can be a gamma spike of realization at the same time as being in the deep and thoughtless spaces of delta.

All these and more combinations of brain activity can be experienced simultaneously in yoga nidrā, because it is a series of cyclical processes that sometimes overlap. This is very useful in terms of managing stress, because it can help us integrate many different levels and types of experiences while we rest. In the relaxed state of yoga nidrā, we can observe all these different states playing out.

▶ Need to know

I want to train myself to stay alert for the whole practice. What can I do to stop myself from falling asleep?

The easiest way to stop yourself from falling asleep during the practice is to be well rested before you begin. So be sure you are getting sufficient sleep, and perhaps do two yoga nidrā practices in a row. During the second one, you will probably stay awake. If your feet are a little cooler than the rest of the body, it can be hard to fall asleep, so perhaps take off your socks or stick your feet out from under the covers. It can also be helpful to rest forearms vertically, with elbows on the ground and hands in the air. In this position, if you fall asleep the forearm will drop and wake you up as it falls in contact with the body or the floor.

How yoga nidrā resources our resilience to manage stress

Experiences of chronic and acute stress are not simply mental experiences. Stress is experienced in all five dimensions of being: our physical body, our vitality, our mental and emotional responses, and our intuitive capacity. We can experience very strong physical reactions to stressful thoughts, and this is precisely why yoga nidrā can be especially helpful in relieving stress. In yoga nidrā, we cycle through multiple cognitive, physical, emotional, and intuitive experiences.

Because yoga nidrā is a cyclical process not a linear journey, it is perfectly normal to cycle through the same set of brain-wave states repeatedly, or sometimes even to get a bit stuck, like a washing machine repeating a rinse cycle. It can all be part of the process, especially if we are feeling stressed. But with practice, we can learn to ease ourselves out of the stressed places and back to alpha zone, or to drop down into theta or delta with a conscious breath or two.

Resilience enables us to sustain our balanced capacity to respond in the face of stressful challenge. We cannot always control what is going on around us, but we can manage our own responses. Yoga nidrā resources our resilience, not only by enabling us to relax to very deep levels where both rest and healing can occur, but also because it gives us time and space to welcome insight and self-awareness.

As we recognize our response to different brain-wave states and other functions in the relaxed space of yoga nidrā, it is easy to do the very simple breath processes that enhance relaxation or help us drop out of states where we feel anxious or stressed. With practice, we can become skilled in evoking or avoiding these states as they arise in the less relaxed space of daily life. We can use familiar, simple techniques as remedies when we meet stressors, and we can also cultivate a basic level of rested-ness that resources us to manage routine daily stressors.

Daily practice is helpful. Making a little time for regular yoga nidrā recipes keeps us well nourished so our bodies are not hungry for rest. When we are hungry for rest, then stress feels worse, because our resilience is depleted. If we keep feeding our resilience with the nourishing ingredients of yoga nidrā, we are less likely to be overwhelmed by the stress of everyday challenges, and we will have the resources to respond well when big, surprising stresses or shocks show up.

As we become more familiar with simple processes of relaxing into yoga nidrā, we learn to settle ourselves, regulating our nervous system's stress responses. This is a gentle and gradual process. With repetition, our bodies and minds learn what it feels like to return to the relaxed state. In this place, even if we encounter stressful thoughts, we learn to recognize their effect on us. When we are in the state of yoga nidrā, we can gently use our breath and our relaxed attention to direct changes in brain-wave activity. We can calm ourselves down, invite insight and inspiration, slow thinking, stop thinking, and, as we discovered in the last chapter, send ourselves off to sleep.

Serving suggestion: Morning nidrā to start the day less stressed

Stress is more difficult to cope with when we're tired. There are times when sleep deprivation or disruption is unavoidable. Yoga nidrā can offset increased anxiety and stress caused by lack of sleep when we're caring for elderly or sick relatives, small children and babies, or when we're working night shifts, meeting tight deadlines, or traveling long-haul. Yoga nidrā makes the most of whatever hours of sleep are realistically possible, helping you to cope better with stress.

Initially, it may seem like an additional stress to add yoga nidrā to a long list of daily tasks. But it's worth making time for a super-short yoga nidrā at the start of the day. Doing nidrā *before* getting out of bed in the morning supports your capacity to deal with whatever challenges may arise.

1. Simply set the alarm 21 minutes before you need to get up, and then do a short nidrā.

2. Alternatively, set the alarm 90 minutes *plus* 21 minutes before your usual wake-up time. Then you can do the short yoga nidrā and drop back to sleep again. Because each sleep cycle is approximately 90 minutes long, this combination gives the added benefit of yoga nidrā, *plus* what feels like a whole additional extra sleep. This doubly resources your resilience, whatever stresses the day may throw at you.

Breathing away stress and pain in yoga nidrā

A long exhale can be a powerful antidote to stress and pain. When we breathe out, we release tension. There are many specific breathing techniques designed to manage different types of pain,[34] but often, the simplest practices, like the ones described earlier, are most potent. They are powerful because we don't have to think too much about them. They arise easily because they are natural patterns of breathing. When we place these simple ingredients in the recipe of yoga nidrā, they can become even more potent than if we simply do them in seated meditation. This is because, in yoga nidrā, we enter a state of trance, and the restorative powers of the breath are more readily received.

Because the body is so deeply relaxed in yoga nidrā, and because these breathing practices are so simple and natural, it is possible to feel as if we can 'breath away' pain, or at least change our relationship to pain. Pain, like stress, is carried in the body and perceived by the mind. There is a close relationship between tension and pain. When we are tense and stressed, our experience of pain is intensified.[35] Learning to regulate our own nervous systems in yoga nidrā, we can change our relationship to bodily sensation through relaxation.

Special recipe: Breathing away stress and pain in yoga nidrā

This is the simplest practice of all.

1. Settling into the practice of yoga nidrā, notice any areas of stress or pain.

2. Inhale and carry your attention into just one area of stress or pain.

3. Exhale with the conscious intention of releasing that stress or pain.

You can use this process in every process of yoga nidrā, or at any other time.

Nidrista story: Easing menstrual pain with yoga nidrā

Many women and menstruators experience severe pain around menstruation, and there is often mental and emotional distress during pre-menstruation. Although the natural physiological process of healthy menstruation is not necessarily painful, the stressful shame and tension surrounding the need to hide the process, or to behave as if it is not happening, can profoundly exacerbate experiences of pain. Yoga nidrā can help relieve both the stress around menstruation and the experience of pain during the bleed.

Anita had spent 20 years experiencing extreme menstrual pain. When she began to do yoga nidrā, she was doubtful that it could make any difference. After two months of daily practice, she experienced her first ever pain-free period. 'My body was in a different place this month,' she explained. 'The yoga nidrā changed every aspect of the experience.' One of the main reasons why regular yoga nidrā is so effective in the relief of stress and pain around menstruation is because the practice enables deep rest during all the other parts of the cycle. A well-rested body is better equipped to handle the physiological demands of monthly menstruation without causing pain. In the resources section, you'll find links to yoga nidrā recordings that are specially designed to support menstrual health.

The special ingredients in this chapter enhance yoga nidrā's capacity to restore rhythmic, natural cycles of physiological and emotional functions in our body mind. This can help us become more balanced in our response to stress, better able to manage pain, and more resilient in the face of the many challenges, painful encounters, injustices, and sufferings that we may experience as humans.

But life is not all suffering and pain. We also have capacity to experience joy and to be filled with boundless vitality and delightful creativity. All these cycles, of suffering and joy, of stress and flowing creativity, can coexist, or circle around each other, in very close proximity, just like in the labyrinth:

When you think you are circling outward, at the next turn, you find yourself in the center. These cyclic paradoxes are the heart of yoga nidrā and power its capacity to sustain and boost energy and creativity, as we'll explore in the next chapter.

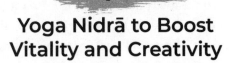

Chapter 13

Yoga Nidrā to Boost Vitality and Creativity

*solutions are small rabbits
in the headlights of our thoughts
frozen into terror by the vehicles we drive
they dash into their burrows if we rush at them too fast –
yoga nidrā lets them gather
so solutions multiply*

The cyclical processes of yoga nidrā can help restore the rhythms of human health and creativity. This chapter shares three simple practical yoga nidrā recipes to boost vitality and nourish a variety of creative cycles. You'll learn how to integrate open intentions within the practice of yoga nidrā to solve problems. You'll also learn some special ingredients for improving dream recall as a tool for boosting energy and creative powers.

The theory behind all these techniques is deeply rooted in the earth-based Indigenous worldview of the Indian yogis and ancient goddess worshippers who first identified the state of yoga nidrā, so this chapter also provides a reminder of just how vital this perspective is to the use of yoga nidrā to enhance your energy cycles.

Energy moves in cycles

Our vitality and creativity are cyclical. If we want to cultivate either capacity, we need to recognize that they move in natural cycles. There will be surges of abundance and quietly ebbing tides when we need to rest and recuperate. These experiences of rhythmicity are an intrinsic part of the creative process, and respect for these cycles is the foundation of vitality. Yoga nidrā helps us learn to recognize the turning tides, know when to power ahead with creative projects or high-energy activities and when to take a break, or put the computer to sleep and take a nap ourselves. This wise and kindly discernment permits us to welcome ourselves just as we are, whatever happens. It is this self-acceptance that boosts vitality and creativity. Simply put, we free up energy when we stop fighting the cyclic processes of life.

The cyclic process of yoga nidrā can support different stages of creative cycles, including inspiration, development, manifestation, and editing. Flashes of inspiration often arise during and after yoga nidrā. Because it is easy to forget such flashes, it is advisable to keep a notebook handy, or other means of recording your inspirational insights, and to make a habit of noting down any inspirations soon after your yoga nidrā process.

▶ *Need to know*

I heard yoga nidrā was good for problem-solving. How does that work?

Because yoga nidrā enables us to let go of our usual patterns of cognitive thought, it can be a highly effective means to innovate and solve problems. The different components of the practice provide many tasks for our thinking mind, and while the conscious mind is busily engaged with these activities, it can free up our unconscious to connect to surprising solutions. We can deliberately state the nature of the problem at the beginning of yoga nidrā (ingredient 3) and invite solutions to arrive by the end of the practice. Sometimes, answers turn up later when we are dreaming, driving the car, or cooking dinner. To capture solutions that might come up as a result of yoga nidrā practice, be sure to write down or record any ideas that arise.

Yoga nidrā can also bring clarity for whittling down, editing, or cutting. Even a brief practice can refresh flagging energy levels and enable you to continue working with diligence and enthusiasm if you are in for the long haul, or perhaps have a deadline looming. Although yoga nidrā practice can often help get creative cycles flowing again in stagnant periods, it also fosters our capacity to distinguish between times of genuine stagnation and periods of gestation, when ideas are growing even though it appears nothing is happening. Yoga nidrā can help us recognize and respect these times as crucial parts of the creative process.

Mystics and scientists concur

Different stages of creative cycles thrive in different states of consciousness. According to yogic philosophy, there are three everyday states of consciousness: waking; dreaming; and deep, dreamless sleep. Beyond these is a secret, fourth state – an experience of pure awareness accessible by meditation and yoga nidrā. The Irish Nobel Laureate poet William Butler Yeats, who had a lifelong scholarly and personal interest in Indian philosophy and liminal states of consciousness, elegantly describes this fourth state as the state 'where the soul, purified of all that is not it, comes into possession of its own timelessness.'[36]

Experiences of these four states are not constant, but rhythmic. We move in cycles from one to another, and yoga nidrā grants access to the places where the different states meet.

Recipe:
Yoga nidrā for cultivating creative focus and vitality

1. Focus attention upon the movement of breath when you settle into yoga nidrā. Feel as if the whole body is breathing. Welcome the current focus of your energies (creative work, relationship, business project) as your intention for your practice (ingredient 3).

2. Be aware of the whole body breathing, and welcome every part, sending breath into all joints, bones, and organs as you carry your awareness around the body in ingredient 4.

3. When you come to ingredient 5, let your attention settle on one single point in the body (perhaps the heart center, or the place between the eyebrows) and then, as you exhale, let your whole awareness rest at that single point.

4. As you inhale, carry your awareness to the periphery, as if the whole body is breathing. As you exhale, carry the awareness back into the single point.

5. Alternate between the single point and the whole body as you breathe.

6. Can you hold awareness of the single point and the whole body at the same time?

7. Can this holding of concentration be effortless? Then can you let it go? Make space for creativity and vital energy to be in the places within and between the single point and the whole body.

8. When you move your attention to the next ingredient, let your effortless concentration rest upon whatever the current focus of your energy is – and let it nourish you.

9. As you complete your yoga nidrā, awaken with a curiosity to discover which aspects of this practice will travel with you into alertness.

▶ Need to know

What's the connection between yoga nidrā and intuition?

Stress and tension can disconnect us from intuitive knowing. Because yoga nidrā relaxes every dimension of being, it invites restfulness into the physical body and mental and emotional processes, while supporting a relaxed connection to sensory awareness and optimizing distribution of energy within bodily systems like blood circulation and digestion. When all these systems enter a relaxed state, it is possible to become more aware of the inner world of intuitive insights that might go unnoticed in daily life. Simply put, the capacity for intuitive knowing is always present, and yoga nidrā can create the conditions to rediscover connection to that intuition.

Special ingredient:
Nasal flows to optimize vital energy

Optimal vitality grows from respect for cyclical wisdom. There is a special cycle of the breath in the nostrils that ancient yogins recognized, and recent scientists also observe – every 90 minutes, the nasal flow shifts from one nostril to the other.[37] The left nostril is associated with more lunar, creative energy, the right nostril with more solar, fiery vitality.

Different energies are suited for different purposes. Next time you prepare to practice yoga nidrā, take a moment to check which nostril breath is naturally flowing. By raising your hand to your nose and deliberately exhaling, you can feel which nostril is more open. Choose to optimize the vital energy supporting your current activities.

❖ To support the fire of the digestive process, logical thinking, and analysis, open the right nostril by resting on the left side.

❖ To cultivate a creative flow of dreamy creative energy, or when you sleep at night, the optimal energy flow is in the left nostril, so rest along the right side and notice expansion in the left nostril.

✦ You can also optimize flow in either nostril by bringing pressure into the opposite armpit – right nostril opens with pressure in left armpit and vice versa.

✦ To cultivate balance between left and right nostril flow, become aware of the little triangle of breath moving in the nose – up both nostrils to eyebrow center and down with every breath. Notice breath moving in both sides. This awareness can be invited into ingredients 2, 3, 7, and 8. You can also use nasal flow as the focus for ingredient

Yoga nidrā recipe for dream incubation

in our resting
within dream states
let us feel these other worlds
that are hidden in the brightness –
invisible to thought –
in activity and striving
we are not able to see
vivid clarity of dream state
that is waiting for our pause –
to come into focus

Dream-state inspiration seeds many creative projects, in life, business, science, and the arts. We can incubate dream fragments in yoga nidrā. The fragments can be nighttime dreams or daydreams, or may be a business project or holiday plan. The fragment might be a dream you have forgotten that you wish you could remember, it could be an idea you have for the next step in your current creative work, or a blue-sky solution to a relationship problem you are facing.

Whatever it is, here are three simple steps to let yoga nidrā help your dream grow.

1. Write or draw the essence of your dream fragment: notes, a rough sketch, a few words, a doodle – it doesn't have to be a work of art so long as it makes sense to you. Bring this image or words into your mind and heart as you settle into yoga nidrā. Invite it to become the third ingredient of yoga nidrā: your intention.

2. When you come to the sixth section of the yoga nidrā, simply inquire: What next? And be curious about what arises either as an image or a felt sense.

3. When you come to the seventh ingredient of yoga nidrā – savoring intent – invite whatever has arisen in the sixth to be present for you. Be curious to sense how it might feel if you had *already* realized the whole dream. At the end of the practice, make notes.

In this chapter, you've savored some of the special yoga nidrā flavors that boost energy and support creative cycles. What's next?

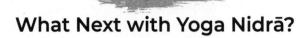

What Next with Yoga Nidrā?

may these nidrā times of listening
empower us to know –
the quiet stillness of our rest
is potent medicine

Congratulations!

If you've got this far, you're already familiar with the nine ingredients of yoga nidrā and have tasted some of the many flavors of yogic sleep. Maybe you have also begun making your own recordings or recalling the sequence of ingredients in your favorite recipes. Now you're ready to step toward the freedom of a personal practice of yoga nidrā that responds to your changing needs.

This chapter offers practical tips for practicing yoga nidrā on the road and shares next steps for your practice of *wild* and *natural* yoga nidrā. Our final gift to you is yoga nidrā in the stars.

Yoga nidrā on the road

Yoga nidrā is a great traveling companion. Travel time can be the perfect opportunity to listen to yoga nidrā recordings on headphones or to self-guide your practice. Be sure to choose a recording that will finish well before you reach your destination or set your timer to give you plenty of time to gather your belongings before you reach your station or deplane. Practicing yoga nidrā on long-haul flights can reduce tiredness on arrival and reduce the impact of jetlag. The trick is to set your timepiece to the time zone of the destination as you buckle up and do back-to-back nidrā as you fly.

Note: It is not safe to listen to yoga nidrā while driving or biking. Never do this. The practice of yoga nidrā guides awareness within. If you are driving or biking, you need all your wits about you, fully attentive to the presence of other road users so that you do not cause an accident. However, if you've parked and are taking a break, yoga nidrā can help increase alertness, which can aid safer driving.

Wild nidrā

may our nidrā time of listening enable us to hear
the patient whispering of these trees
whose rooted voices speak
the wisdom buried in the earth

Once you can navigate into and out of the practice in your familiar yoga nidrā nest at home, you can explore the wonders of *wild* nidrā – yoga nidrā anywhere, made with whatever ingredients you find. This is the next step from simply listening to your favorite nidrā recipes outside.

Wild nidrā invites you to listen to whatever sounds you hear and integrate them into your own experience of yoga nidrā. Eventually, you don't need words. Let the contact between your body and the earth root your settling into stillness. Let the feeling of sunlight on your skin guide movements of awareness around the body. Let the sound of wind in the trees call your intention alive and let the song of running water lull you deeply into yoga nidrā. Perhaps birdsong will call you back at the end of the practice, or maybe a dog will bark and awaken you. Be sure you are totally familiar with the externalization and finishing stages of yoga nidrā before trying this. Being ready for anything, as the state of yoga nidrā arising wordlessly is the essence of wild nidrā. To begin with, it can be helpful to have a sparsely guided nidrā practice to support this wordless process, and there is a 'Welcoming wild nidrā' (audio track 11.0) to listen to if that feels useful (see listing on page 2).

Freedom from the known: Natural yoga nidrā

How simple can this be? Since yoga nidrā is a naturally arising state of human consciousness, it is no surprise that, when we begin to cultivate our capacity to enter this state, it may simply begin to show up by itself. This is the implicit paradox at the heart of the yoga nidrā labyrinth.

All it takes is practice, curiosity, and a willingness to welcome what arises.

Simply making space and time to rest in yoga nidrā most days, through listening to recordings or self-guiding practice, we remind ourselves how it feels to rest in yoga nidrā. A pleasant side effect of this conscious effort is the unbidden arrival of yoga nidrā in daily life. You may find small flashes of yoga nidrā states begin to show up at moments when you least expect them. Perhaps you are dozing off one afternoon or pausing to notice clouds as you take out the recycling, or maybe in a lull in conversation you simply drop into a receptive restful space. Simply allow yourself to receive these gifts as fruits of your practice and welcome natural yoga nidrā in momentary everyday lucidity. Initially, it can be supportive to have an almost wordless nidrā with time checks to encourage the naturally arising state, so we have made a 'Welcoming wordless yoga nidrā' (audio track 12.0) for you to hear if that seems helpful (see listing on page 2).

Yoga nidrā in the stars

An exquisite traditional Himalayan practice of yoga nidrā places tiny blue stars at 61 points in a journey of awareness around the body. Next time you settle to self-guide your yoga nidrā process, invite a glimpse or a sense of sparkling stars in all the places in your body that you visit in your chosen rotation of consciousness. Let the pairs of opposites be the constellations of these stars and the spaces between them. Rest in yoga nidrā, simultaneously aware of the spaces in the night sky of the body, and the places where the stars sparkle. Enjoy your cosmic yogic sleep and be sure to externalize fully before completing the practice. If you prefer, you can listen to this process on audio track 13.0 (see listing on page 2).

Conclusion

Cycling Back to Where We Began

how simple would you like it?
how easy can it be –
to stop what you are doing and lie down upon the floor?
this tiny act is all it takes
to turn your world around
to wake up to the taste of restful being
here and now

A s this book is an easy beginner's guide, we haven't explored many of the more profound implications of yoga nidrā in relation to the nature of reality, freedom, death, or consciousness. Neither have we discussed in depth the extraordinary ancient histories of yoga nidrā, the troubling politics of commercially appropriating Indian spiritual practices and Indigenous traditions, or the problematic power structures in contemporary organizations that teach trademarked methods of yoga nidrā.

If you want to take your journey with yoga nidrā further and understand more about these topics, we invite you to check out *Nidrā Shakti: The Power of Rest – An Illustrated Encyclopaedia of Yoga Nidrā*, which offers a comprehensive and multilevel presentation of yoga nidrā and includes 127 transcripts of live, improvised yoga nidrā practices.

However, from this easy guide, you already have a thorough grounding in the basics of yoga nidrā. Even the simplest practice of yoga nidrā can help restore rhythmic, natural cycles of life and reconnect you to vitality, well-being, and inspiration. In this book, we've laid out a nourishing range of ingredients for your own personal yoga nidrā recipes.

Above and beyond all the other things that it can offer, yoga nidrā brings us home to a state of rest and self-acceptance. We all need to rest to thrive, and without proper rest, life is so much more of a struggle. Yoga nidrā not only helps us get high-quality rest any time we need, but it also empowers us to understand the workings of our own consciousness.

> *all it takes is 20 minutes to be horizontal here –*
> *all it takes is lying quietly*
> *backing down*
> *and stepping back*

Regular practice of yoga nidrā helps us navigate the different states of awareness we encounter day and night so that we can become more fully lucid in our life – awake, asleep, or dreaming. This is truly life-changing at every level. Recall some of the real-life improvements and changes experienced effortlessly by the nidristas mentioned in this book: from the tiny daily breakthroughs to the total transformations; from ending irritating bad habits, such as nail-biting, to resolving deep-seated phobias, such as fear of flying; from effortlessly letting go of harmful addictions to effectively managing acute conditions, such as cancer, or chronic complaints, such as insomnia.

Many thousands of people all over the world have already experienced these benefits of yoga nidrā, and some have transformed their experiences of deep pain or grief. What they all have in common is not that they are super-devoted practitioners whose lives revolve around yoga nidrā, but just that they made little spaces to pause and welcome the possibility that their natural rhythmic cycles could be restored to health and vitality through the simple practice of yoga nidrā.

The naturally arising yoga nidrā state is an extraordinary gift – a way to rest and encounter the paradoxes of human experience, to be nourished and refreshed, inspired, and relieved of sufferings large and small, even just to remember how to sleep. Through the very simple practice of becoming aware of the processes of falling asleep, and through the act of effortlessly meditating upon this nightly experience, we can welcome deeply healing states of being into our everyday lives, inviting possibilities to become conscious of how we navigate human challenges of every kind.

As we prepared this book, we had the privilege to work with people using yoga nidrā to transform their lives through rest, healing, creativity, and personal breakthroughs. A nurse, who nearly died from Covid after becoming infected when working in the intensive care unit of her local hospital, has used yoga nidrā to help her recover respiratory function and overcome her fear of death. A professional musician whose crippling performance anxiety was threatening his capacity to play music is now using yoga nidrā to manage his stress levels so he can work again. A woman who had experienced multiple miscarriages and failed IVF attempts used yoga nidrā to support the conception, gestation, and birth of a healthy child. A burned-out doctor with debilitating depression and anxiety regained his confidence through daily yoga nidrā practice, stepped sideways into a different field of medicine, and awoke to discover that he loved his job. A young forestry worker, who'd nearly died in a serious car accident, resolved more than a decade of post-traumatic stress and painful digestive disorders by simply lying down and listening to the yoga nidrā practice specially created for her in one-to-one yoga nidrā sessions.

Often, people come to yoga nidrā when they feel they are at the end of the road, when they have given up hope. They are then astonished to discover just how potent the simple act of restful meditation upon the act of falling asleep can be. We have barely begun to understand the extraordinary and limitless healing potential of this practice.

At our teacher and facilitator trainings, we often reassure people that it doesn't matter if you can remember whatever you heard during yoga nidrā. What matters is that you settle into a space where you can welcome intuitive guidance and let your body's natural, rhythmic cycles restore and recalibrate. When we consciously choose to let go and make space for such effortless resettling in our lives, we reconnect to the power of life itself, and many things that felt difficult seem to become possible.

When we share yoga nidrā, in person or online, we remind people that this is inherently a practice of conscious surrender into wholeness through the experience of being received and held. When we simply feel how it is to be welcomed in our horizontal surrender by the surface beneath us, when we find ourselves awake and asleep at the same time, witnessing our own state of simply being, we can discover that relinquishing the drive always to be 'doing' gives us abundant resources to become better at simply 'being.' We can come home to the generous nurture of Earth herself and return, after our practice, refreshed and nourished, better able to be kinder to ourselves and to others.

We invite you to make a little space on most days to welcome the humble, generous, and natural practice of yoga nidrā into your life, and to observe the shifts and changes that can unfold effortlessly.

In the next section, you'll find a wealth of resources to accompany you on your further adventures with yoga nidrā, but you already have everything you need to make this practice your own. Remember that there is no way to do yoga nidrā wrong, because there is nothing to *do*. Be guided by intuitive wisdoms that arise as your body drifts toward the threshold of sleep. In the space of yoga nidrā, we invite you to follow your heart: It knows the way home to yourself.

Thank you for reading. Thank you for resting.

With great respect and love, we send warm wishes for your well-being and blessings for your practice of yoga nidrā.

Uma Dinsmore-Tuli and Nirlipta Tuli

Midsummer Solstice 2021

A closing yoga nidrā poem

the challenge here within us
is to make the choice to stop –
to receive the restful nurture that is waiting if we pause
to be in a place of quietness and to rest a moment more
to receive yoga nidrā as we lie upon the floor –
it looks like nothing happens
but the taste of resting here
is the flavor of deep nurture that reconnects us all
to the rhythmic vital cycles that nourish all of life.

A blessing for all yoga nidristas

We tend now to the inner light that shines
within these hearts,
We nurture now the embers that can warm
a deeper trust.
We rest and know that in this pause,
Our earth upon this land,
We invite reconnection to the pulse of all that lives.

And through this reconnection,
We do honor life herself:
The earth and sky, the fire and air,
The space that holds us all.
We choose to rest and honor life
And afterward arise
to face the world, and all that lives,
with heart and soul renewed.

References

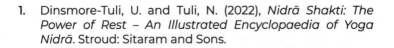

1. Dinsmore-Tuli, U. and Tuli, N. (2022), *Nidrā Shakti: The Power of Rest – An Illustrated Encyclopaedia of Yoga Nidrā*. Stroud: Sitaram and Sons.

2. Labyrinths exist in many cultures globally. This composite model was specially made to illustrate the nine-part process of Total Yoga Nidrā. Uma first began integrating group yoga nidrā experience with labyrinths in 2016, and this image combines her experience of two labyrinths: the Loop Head Celtic Labyrinth at Pure Camping in Querrin, County Clare, Ireland, and an ancient Indian birthing yantra 'Chakra Vyahu,' painted by Nirlipta Tuli in 1998 to support the birth of our first son.

3. The original version of this rhythmic yoga nidrā practice entitled 'Yoga Nidrā Lullaby' first appeared in *Nidrā Shakti: The Power of Rest – An Illustrated Encyclopaedia of Yoga Nidrā*. This specially simplified version has been adapted for *Yoga Nidrā Made Easy* by the authors. Audio recordings freely available at www.yoganidranetwork.org.

4. Coburn, T. B. (1991), *Encountering the Goddess: A Translation of the Devī-Māhātmya and a Study of Its Interpretation*. Albany: State University of New York Press.

5. Coburn, T. B. (1984), *Devī-Māhātmya: The Crystallization of the Goddess Tradition*. Delhi: Motilal Banarsidass.

6. Pattanaik, D. (2011), 'Lakshman's wife goes to sleep.': devdutt.com/articles/indian-mythology/ramayana/lakshmans-wife-goes-to-sleep.html [Accessed Feb 21, 2022]

7. If you are interested in the many other fascinating stories of the goddess Yoga Nidrā Shakti, we have included them in *Nidrā Shakti: The Power of Rest – An Illustrated Encyclopaedia of Yoga Nidrā*.

8. Stiles, M. (2001), *Yoga Sutras of Patanjali*. San Francisco: Red Wheel/Weiser.

9. Rama, S. (1982), *Enlightenment Without God: Commentary on Māṇḍukya Upaniṣad*. Himalayan International Institute of Yoga Science and Philosophy.

10. *The Hatha Yoga Pradipika* (1972), Madras: The Theosophical Society. https://archive.org/details/hathayogapradipika/mode/2up?view=theater [Accessed October 12, 2021]

11. Campaign document downloads: 'Compilation of Evidence' available at https://yonishakti.co/the-movement

12. Tuli, N., Dinsmore-Tuli, U. (2021), 'In Defence of the Practice of Yoga Nidrā', www.yoganidranetwork.org/blog/defence-practice-yoga-nidra [Accessed November 12, 2021]

13. The Nap Ministry (2021), 'How will you be useless to capitalism today?', https://thenapministry.wordpress.com/ [Accessed November 12, 2021]

14. Heavy eye pillows prevent rapid eye movement (REM). Use a lighter pillow, or none, if you want to permit REM, or if you find it hard to focus after yoga nidrā.

15. Miller, R. (2015), *The iRest Program for Healing PTSD: A Proven-Effective Approach to Using Yoga Nidrā Meditation and Deep Relaxation Techniques to Overcome Trauma.* Oakland: New Harbinger.

16. Lucy Crisfield, 'Samkalpa', www.originalwisdom.co.uk/sa%e1%b9%81kalpa-bringing-the-mother-of-the-gods-to-court [Accessed November 12, 2021]

17. Over 40 personal accounts of using yoga nidrā to support healing recovery, including after serious brain injury, are documented in *Nidrā Shakti: The Power of Rest – An Illustrated Encyclopaedia of Yoga Nidrā.*

18. Boyes, D. (1973), *Le Yoga Du Sommeil Eveillé.* France: Editions Epi.

19. For a useful practical explanation of how to use yoga nidrā to manage addictions and bad habits, see Kamini Desai's *Yoga Nidrā: the Art of Transformational Sleep* (2016).

20. Walker, M. (2017), *Why We Sleep: Unlocking the Power of Sleep and Dreams*, New York: Allen Lane.

21. NHS, 'Why Lack of Sleep is Bad for Your Health', www.nhs.uk/live-well/sleep-and-tiredness/why-lack-of-sleep-is-bad-for-your-health [Accessed October 11, 2021]

22. The global prevalence of sleep disorders has officially been identified as an epidemic. Sanders, N. 'Sleep disorders, the Silent Epidemic?', www.sleepstation.org.uk/articles/sleep-science/sleep-epidemic [Accessed October 11, 2021]

23. Eighty-three percent of people with depression are insomniacs. The Good Body (2018), 'Just How Little Are We Sleeping?', www.thegoodbody.com/insomnia-statistics [Accessed October 11, 2021]

24. Sharpe, E., Lacombe, A., et al. (2021), 'A Closer Look at Yoga Nidrā: Sleep Lab Protocol', *International Journal of Yoga Therapy*, 10, 17761/2021-D-20-00004.

25. Green, E.et al. (1970), 'Voluntary Control of Internal States: Psychological and Physiological', *Journal of Transpersonal Psychology*, 1, 1–26; Kjaer, T.W. et al. (2002), 'Increased Dopamine Tone During Meditation-Induced Change of Consciousness', *Cognitive Brain Research*, 13, 225–259; Mandlik, V. et al. (2009), 'Effect of Yoga Nidrā on EEG', Unpublished report. Nasik, Maharashtra, India: Yoga Vidya Gurukul University.

26. The distinction between REM and NREM (non-rapid eye movement) sleep was made in 1959 by Michel Jouvet, who coined the phrase 'paradoxical sleep.'

27. Ekirch, A. R. (2006), *At Day's Close: Night in Times Past*. New York: W.W. Norton & Company.

28. Association of Anaesthetists, 'Fight Fatigue Resources Pack', https://anaesthetists.org/Home/Wellbeing-support/ Fatigue/-Fight-Fatigue-download-our-information-packs [Accessed October 11, 2021]

29. Sanders, N. 'Sleep disorders, the Silent Epidemic?', www. sleepstation.org.uk/articles/sleep-science/sleep-epidemic [Accessed October 11, 2021]

30. 'Sleep Well with Yoga Nidrā' and 'Yoga Nidrā for a Good Night's Sleep' by Nirlipta Tuli are good examples of nidrā designed to ease you into sleep and leave you resting there. Available on www.yoganidranetwork.org.

31. Connor J. et al. (2002), 'Driver Sleepiness and Risk of Serious Injury', *BMJ*, 324,1125.

32. Shannahoff-Khalsa, David et al. (2001), 'Ultradian Rhythms of Alternating Cerebral Hemispheric EEG Dominance Are Coupled to Rapid Eye Movement and Non-Rapid Eye Movement Stage 4 Sleep in Humans', *Sleep Medicine*, 2, 2001.

33. Kumar, K. & Pandya, P. (2012). 'A Study on the Impact on ESR Level through Yogic Relaxation Technique Yoga Nidra', *Indian Journal of Traditional Knowledge*, 11, 358–361.

34. For a range of effective breath techniques to manage pain in childbirth and postnatal recovery, see Dinsmore-Tuli, U. (2006) *Mother's Breath: A definitive Guide to Yoga Breathing, Sound and Awareness Practices During Pregnancy, Birth, Postnatal Recovery and Mothering*. Stroud: Sitaram and Sons; for menstrual pain management see Dinsmore-Tuli, U. (2016) *Yoni Shakti*. Stroud: Sitaram and Sons.

35. The 'fear-tension-pain' cycle was first described by British doctor Grantley Dick-Read, who observed that fear of pain would lead to physical tension in anticipation of it, which would lead to heightened sensations of pain.

36. Yeats, W. B. (1994), *Later Essays by Yeats, W. B. 1865–1939*. New York: Charles Scribner's Sons. Also, Swami, S. P. and Yeats, W.B. (1937), *The Ten Principal Upanishads*. London: Faber.

37. Gronfier, C. et al. (1998), 'Ultradian Rhythms in Pituitary and Adrenal Hormones: Their relations to Sleep', *Sleep Medicine Reviews*, vol. 2, no. 1: 17–29.

Recommended Reading

Andrews, Munya. *Journey into Dreamtime*. Ultimate World Publishing, 2019.

Brody, Karen. *Daring to Rest: Reclaim Your Power with Yoga Nidrā Rest Meditation. A 40 Day Program for Women*. Sounds True, 2017.

Brown, Adrienne Maree. *Pleasure Activism: The Politics of Feeling Good*. AK Press, 2019.

Desai, Kamini. *Yoga Nidrā: The Art of Transformational Sleep: Restore Your Health, Reshape Your Life, and Change Your Destiny*. Lotus Press, 2017.

Dumpert, Jennifer. *Liminal Dreaming: Exploring Consciousness at the Edges of Sleep*. North Atlantic, 2019.

Lusk, Julie. *Yoga Nidrā Meditations: 24 Scripts for True Relaxation*. Llewellyn, 2021.

Magaña, Sergio Ocelocoyotl. *The Toltec Secret: Dreaming Practices of the Ancient Mexicans*. Hay House, 2014.

Miller, Richard. *Yoga Nidrā: A meditative practice for deep relaxation and healing.* Sounds True, 2005.

Morley, Charlie. *Wake Up to Sleep: Five Practices to Transform Stress and Trauma for Peaceful Sleep.* Hay House, 2021.

Naiman, Rubin. *Healing Night: The Science and Spirit of Sleeping, Dreaming and Awakening.* New Moon Media, 2014.

Stanley, Tracee. *Radiant Rest: Yoga Nidrā for Deep Relaxation and Awakened Clarity.* Shambhala, 2021.

Taylor, Sonya Renee. *The Body is Not an Apology: The Power of Radical Self Love.* Berrett-Koehler, 2021.

Walker, Matthew. *Why We Sleep: The New Science of Sleep and Dreams.* Penguin, 2018.

Resources

Further adventures in yoga nidrā

To learn more about the practice, we recommend our comprehensive guide, *Nidrā Shakti: The Power of Rest – An Illustrated Encyclopaedia of Yoga Nidrā*, Sitaram and Sons, 2022.

For more recordings to support your practice of yoga nidrā, please see the following, and more, on our website:

◆ 'Total Yoga Nidrā for the peoples now' – Easy yoga nidrā for everyone to integrate the practice of yoga nidrā into everyday life, including practices to support positive digestion and reduce anxiety. Thirteen audio tracks and seven video chats with Nirlipta Tuli and Uma Dinsmore-Tuli.

◆ 'Sleep well with yoga nidrā' – Online course for insomniacs and all who would like to sleep better, by Nirlipta Tuli.

- ❖ 'Yoni Shakti Well Woman Yoga Therapy Immersion Experience' – Online course with six yoga nidrā tracks to support menstrual and menopausal health, and monthly live webinar support with Uma Dinsmore-Tuli.

- ❖ 'Yoni nidrā' – Yoga nidrā audio album for women's health by Uma Dinsmore-Tuli.

Gifts and gatherings

It's always lovely to hear from readers about your experiences with yoga nidrā, so we warmly invite you to connect with us on social media. We share free, live, online Total Yoga Nidrā co-creative practices on Instagram (@umadinsmoretuli and @yoganidranetwork), on Facebook (@UmaDinsmoretuliPhd), and on our yoga nidrā Facebook community page www.facebook.com/yoganidranetwork.

All the inspiring people whose stories we tell in this book are real. Some are yoga therapy clients and yoga nidrā colleagues, some are our students, and some are teachers we have trained. We met them all through the Yoga Nidrā Network, and we invite you to join us there in our virtual community gathering circles and online learning sanctuary www.yoganidranetwork.org.

Enjoy free, authentic yoga nidrā recordings in 23 different languages on the Yoga Nidrā Network site. Finding trustworthy audio nidrās online can be a bit hit and miss, so this a reliable source of tracks from trusted teachers.

This is also where you can find local facilitators near you for live, in-person sessions, and discover oodles of our yoga nidrā albums, including yoga nidrā for children, for sleep, for women's health, and for everyday use.

All the yoga nidrā verses in this book are harvested from Uma's continuing creative output, which she shares with subscribers in her Patreon circles. For live, online regular co-creative yoga nidrā sessions, nighttime dreamcatcher nidrā slumber parties, monthly lunar nidrā readings, and patron-only sneak previews of the latest yoga nidrā and creative writing work, you can meet up with Uma on her Patreon page: https://www.patreon.com/umadinsmoretuli.

Learning and training together

Much of the material in this book is based on the Yoga Nidrā Network's multilevel trainings in Total Yoga Nidrā, and you are welcome to join us in person and online at one of our many courses and workshops, including:

❖ 'Total Yoga Nidrā Immersion Experience Online' – Stand-alone course, also a prerequisite for our teacher and facilitator training courses.

❖ 'Yoga Nidrā Network Open Circles' – Monthly online gatherings for all facilitators of yoga nidrā.

❖ 'Total Yoga Nidrā Teacher and Facilitator Training Courses" – With Nirlipta Tuli, Uma Dinsmore-Tuli, and Yoga Nidrā Network tutors.

◆ 'Yoni Shakti Well Woman Yoga Therapy for Women's Health' – Online training course with 27 yoga nidrā audio tracks to support women's health, and nine monthly live webinars and classes with Uma Dinsmore-Tuli.

Nidrista resources

Many of the colleagues whose stories are shared in this book offer their own trainings and workshops in yoga nidrā:

◆ Yoli Maya Yeh Joseph's decolonizing grief and healing work: Instagram @yoliyogini

◆ Karen Brody's Daring to Rest method: www. daringtorest.com

◆ Tricia Hersey's Nap Ministry: www.thenapministry. wordpress.com

◆ Collette Carroll's yoga nidrā for recovery from addiction: www.recoverynidra.com

Many ways to practice

There are several popular techniques deriving from the main schools of yoga nidrā, including Tracee Stanley's Radiant Rest, and Rod Stryker's ParaYoga Nidrā, which both derive primarily from Swami Rama's Himalayan Institute approach. Other approaches include Julie Lusk's *Yoga Nidrā for Complete Relaxation and Stress Relief*, and ISHTA (Integrated Science of Hatha, Tantra, and Ayurveda) yoga nidrā.

Index

Exercises and illustrations are in *italics*.

About the Authors

Nirlipta and Uma established the Yoga Nidra Network in 2010 and are coauthors of *Nidrā Shakti: The Power of Rest – An Illustrated Encyclopaedia of Yoga Nidrā* (2022). Their coevolution of Total Yoga Nidrā is an inclusive, ethical, postlineage initiative, *entirely independent* of any affiliation to other yoga institutes. Uma and Nirlipta prize the endogenous arising of natural yoga nidrā as a daily practice and empower others to welcome this potent nourishment into everyday life. Nirlipta and Uma are both certified members of the International Association of Yoga Therapists (CIAYT). They teach together and separately, online and in person, in Europe and around the world.

Yoga nidrā has always been a central feature of their approach to yoga therapy. Teaching yoga since 1989, Nirlipta has an MA in Indian religions, a diploma in clinical hypnotherapy, and a degree in art history. He created all the illustrations for Uma's book *Yoni Shakti: A Woman's Guide to Power and Freedom through Yoga and Tantra* (2014). Uma's PhD is in communications, and she holds two diplomas in yoga therapy. Teaching yoga since 1996, she has been training teachers and yoga therapists internationally since 2003.

Born in Luton to Indian parents in 1964, Nirlipta first encountered yoga in 1987 in HMP Blantyre House. Born in London to an Irish mother and English father in 1965, Uma first encountered yoga while watching *Yoga for Health* on Thames TV in 1969.

Proud to live in Stroud, a funky rural town in the Cotswold Hills of England, Nirlipta and Uma now share their home with six cats and a small Schnauzer. Their three children were all born at home in the Sitaram South London Yoga Centre where, for 10 years, Nirlipta and Uma shared therapeutic yoga and yoga nidrā with thousands of local families. They both share a deep reverence for dreams, Indian food, and the goddess Nidrā Shakti. About much else, they disagree.

We love to hear from you! Do sign up for our newsletter at www.yoganidranetwork.org

Or find us sharing yoga nidrā on the socials:

 @umadinsmoretuli @yoganidranetwork

 @umadinsmoretuliphd and @yoganidranetwork

For poems and seasonal yoga nidrā exclusives head over to Uma's Patreon page www.patreon.com/umadinsmoretuli.

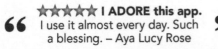

Hay House Podcasts
Bring Fresh, Free Inspiration Each Week!

Hay House proudly offers a selection of life-changing audio content via our most popular podcasts!

Hay House Meditations Podcast

Features your favorite Hay House authors guiding you through meditations designed to help you relax and rejuvenate. Take their words into your soul and cruise through the week!

Dr. Wayne W. Dyer Podcast

Discover the timeless wisdom of Dr. Wayne W. Dyer, world-renowned spiritual teacher and affectionately known as "the father of motivation." Each week brings some of the best selections from the 10-year span of Dr. Dyer's talk show on Hay House Radio.

Hay House Podcast

Enjoy a selection of insightful and inspiring lectures from Hay House Live events, listen to some of the best moments from previous Hay House Radio episodes, and tune in for exclusive interviews and behind-the-scenes audio segments featuring leading experts in the fields of alternative health, self-development, intuitive medicine, success, and more! Get motivated to live your best life possible by subscribing to the free Hay House Podcast.

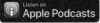

Find Hay House podcasts on iTunes, or visit www.HayHouse.com/podcasts for more info.

HAY HOUSE

Look within

Join the conversation about latest products,
events, exclusive offers and more.

 Hay House

 @HayHouseUK

 @hayhouseuk

We'd love to hear from you!